Books should be returned on or before the
last date stamped below

2 2 MAR 2005

- 7 AUG 2006

2 1 MAR 2012

- 9 MAY 2013

3 0 OCT 2015

1 3 APR 2016

- 7 MAR 2017

hamlyn

aromatherapy
solutions

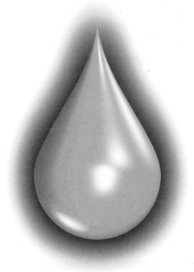

Essential oils to lift the mind, body and spirit

Veronica Sibley

First published in Great Britain in 2003 by
Hamlyn, a division of Octopus Publishing Group Ltd
2–4 Heron Quays, London E14 4JP

Distributed in the United States and Canada by
Sterling Publishing Co., Inc.
387 Park Avenue South, New York, NY 10016–8810

ISBN 0 600 60684 8

A CIP catalogue record for this book is available from the
British Library

Printed and bound in China

10 9 8 7 6 5 4 3 2 1

SAFETY NOTE
This book should not be considered a replacement for
professional medical treatment. A medical practitioner should
be consulted in all matters related to health. While the advice
and information in this book is believed to be accurate and
the step-by-step instructions have been devised to avoid
strain, neither the publisher nor the author can accept legal
responsibility for any injury or illness sustained while
following the exercises and advice included.

Contents

Introduction

Aromatherapy is a gentle but effective method of healing and enhancing the mind, body and spirit through the use of natural oils from aromatic plants, trees and grasses; it provides a valuable alternative to chemical-based medicines. This book explains what these oils are, how they work and how to use them, including an aromatherapy massage section with step-by-step photography. All the common ailments that can benefit from aromatherapy are covered, as is its value in treating emotional and mental problems, with details of the recommended essential oils and how they should be used. Essential oils can also be used in the home and a room-by-room guide shows how to harness the power of plants in your daily life. Finally a directory at the end of the book sets out the properties and uses of all the recommended essential oils and carrier oils.

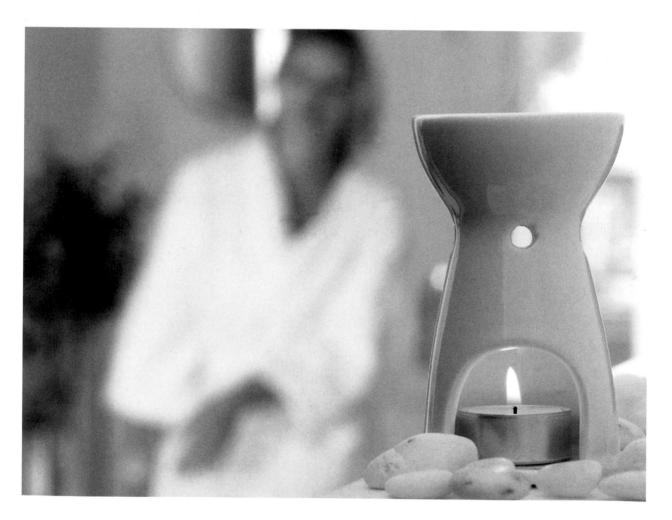

Cautions and sensitivity

Skin-patch test

If you have very sensitive skin or any allergies, it is advisable to test any essential oil or carrier oil before using it. To do this, try the skin-patch test, as follows.

✳ Brush the inside of your lower arm (elbow to wrist) with a soft body-brush.

✳ Apply 2 drops of the essential oil to an antiseptic-free plaster.

✳ Place on the inside of the forearm and leave for 48 hours.

✳ If you are sensitive to plasters, apply oil neat to the skin and cover with micropore and bandage.

Sensitivities to essential oils tend to show up quite quickly, while carrier oil allergies and sensitivities can take several hours to appear. If any redness, swelling or blistering (the latter is rare) occur, this is a positive result, and you should avoid that particular oil.

Treating an adverse reaction

If any adverse reaction does occur, one or more of the following steps should be taken.

✳ Wash the skin gently with fragrance-free soap. This will remove oils from the surface.

✳ Expose the skin to the air (not to sunlight). This will encourage evaporation of some of the oil.

✳ Apply a mild corticosteroid cream, which would be the standard medical approach.

Contraindications

Always check the Directory of essential oils (see pages 116–123) and the Directory of carrier oils (see pages 124–125) for cautions and contraindications before using any oil. The following oils should not be used in the stated instances.

✳ Avoid if taking aspirin, heparin or warfarin: bay.

✳ Avoid if taking paracetamol: fennel.

✳ Avoid during pregnancy: cajuput, camomile (Roman), celery seed, cinnamon leaf, clary sage, fennel, jasmine absolute, juniper berry, lavandin, lavender, spike lavender, marjoram (sweet), myrrh, niaouli, rosemary, tagetes, yarrow.

✳ Avoid use for babies and young children: fennel, may chang, niaouli, peppermint, tagetes.

✳ Avoid use with high blood pressure: rosemary, thyme (red).

✳ Avoid use with fever: lavandin, spike lavender.

✳ Avoid use with epilepsy: fennel, lavandin, spike lavender, rosemary.

✳ Avoid use with liver problems (including alcoholism): fennel, rosemary.

✳ Avoid use with allergies: almond (sweet) carrier oil, wheatgerm carrier oil.

✳ Avoid use with skin sensitivity: citronella, clove, eucalyptus (*E. citriodora*), geranium, manuka, may chang, peppermint, tea tree, thyme (red), ylang ylang.

✳ The following oils are photosensitive or phototoxic – when using them you should keep out of the sun: angelica, bergamot, grapefruit, lemon, lime, tagetes, ylang ylang.

What are essential oils?

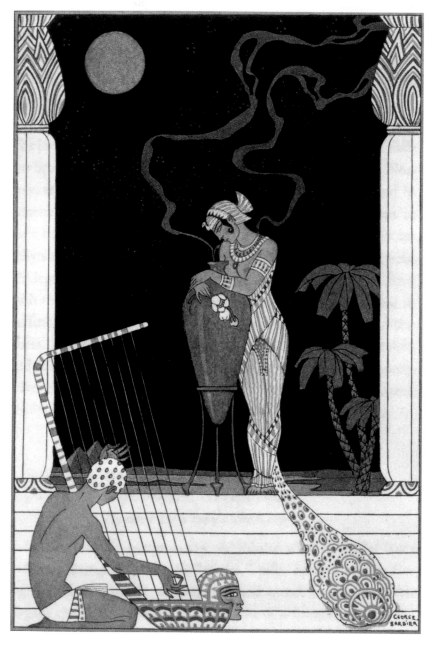

Above 'Egypt', a print from 'The Art of Perfume', published in 1912.

Nature has provided us with a healing agent which can be used to enhance our mind, body and spirit. This healing agent comes in the form of 'essential oils', also sometimes known as 'essences' or 'volatile oils', which are extracted from aromatic plants, trees and grasses. These oils accumulate in the glands or sacs within the fibres of the plant, and it is thought that their function is to aid pollination, help with the survival of the plant and prevent attack from predators.

Essential oils can be found in different parts of the plant:

❋ flowers (lavender and rose)
❋ fruit (lemon)
❋ leaves (eucalyptus)
❋ berries (black pepper)
❋ bark resin (frankincense)
❋ cones (cypress)
❋ heartwood (sandalwood)
❋ rhizomes (ginger)
❋ roots of grass (vetiver)

The orange tree is unusual as it produces three different essential oils, each with differing medicinal properties:

❋ neroli comes from the blossom, and is bittersweet and sedating.
❋ petitgrain comes from the leaves, and is beneficial for the skin.
❋ the rind provides bitter orange, which can help relieve anxiety and worry.

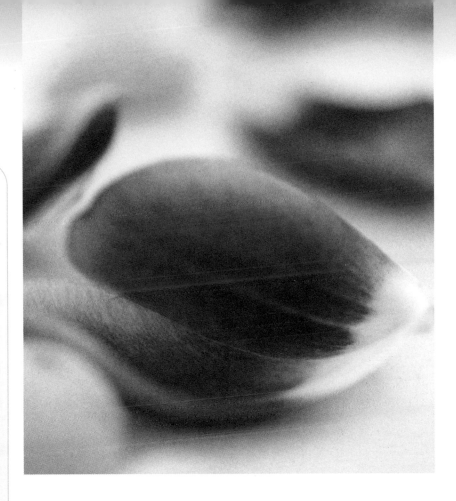

Producing oils

It takes a lot of work to produce a drop of essential oil. Sixty thousand rose blossoms are required to produce 25g (1oz) of rose oil, whereas lavender is easier to obtain and can yield 3 litres (5 pints) of oil from 100kg (220lb) of dried flowers.

Jasmine and rose flowers have to be picked by hand before the sun rises as the heat of the sun will evaporate the essential oil within the petals.

The sandalwood tree must be 30 years old and over 9m (30ft) tall before it can be cut down for distillation.

The wide range of extremes in growing and picking plants is reflected in the price of each essential oil. Jasmine is one of the most expensive – it takes eight million hand-picked jasmine blossoms to produce 1 litre (1¾ pints) of essential oil.

Names of plants

In the Directory of essential oils (pages 116–123), for the plants used in aromatherapy, botanical names (based on Latin) appear as well as English common names. This may seem intimidating, but the botanical names are standard all over the world, unlike common names, and using them therefore eliminates any possible confusion. Every plant has a unique botanical name that is always in two parts. The first is that of the genus and it is always capitalized. The second is the species name, which is always in lower case. Both are always written in italic.

For example, one species of eucalyptus, a common plant in aromatherapy, is called *Eucalyptus* (genus) *globulus* (species). Each species has different properties. For example, *Eucalyptus globulus*, high in oxides and ketones (see page 14), is a good oil for adults who suffer from colds and sinus problems. *Eucalyptus smithii* has oxides but not ketones, making it a safer oil to use for children with colds and sinus problems. *Eucalyptus citriodora*, full of aldehydes (see page 14), is not used for colds, but makes a good insect-repellent.

If in any doubt, always check the Directory (pages 116–123) to make sure you are using the correct oil.

Where do oils come from?

Essential oils come from all over the world. Camomile, peppermint, rose and yarrow originate in England; eucalyptus, niaouli and tea tree in Australia; cedarwood in the USA; ylang ylang and ravensara in Madagascar; petitgrain in Paraguay; cardamom in Guatemala; ginger in China; sandalwood in India; tarragon and lavender in France. The same species of plant grown in different countries under different soil and altitude conditions will produce oils that differ in their chemical make-up and therapeutic properties.

Thyme (*Thymus vulgaris*) grown at high altitude will produce a high alcohol content because the plant is grown in the sun and light, but if grown at low altitude and in darker conditions will produce phenols (see page 14) within the plant. A high percentage of phenols within the oil is aggressive and can be an irritant to

the skin. Both of these oils are beneficial for colds and flu, but *Thymus vulgaris* grown at high altitude is considered safer to use because of the lower phenol content.

Lavender (*Lavandula angustifolia*) grown in the South of France has a high ester (see page 14) content, which is soothing and healing for the skin; lavender grown in Bulgaria has a higher alcohol content, which has good astringent properties and is cleansing for the skin; lavender grown in England has a sweeter smell than that grown in France, where the aroma of the oil is more heady and deep.

How is the oil extracted?

The essential oil is extracted from the plant by a variety of means. The most common are steam distillation, expression and maceration.

✳ **Steam distillation** involves placing the plant material in water, which is then brought to the boil. The steam containing the volatile essential oil is run through a cooler, where it condenses, and the liquid distillate is gathered. The essential oil appears as a thin film on top of the liquid. The essential oil is then separated from the water.

✳ **Citrus oil** is expressed rather than distilled. Within the citrus fruits, the essential oil is located in little sacs just under the surface of the rind. The oil needs to be squeezed out, and this is achieved by letting the fruit roll over a conveyer that has small needles coming out, piercing the little oil pockets in the citrus rind. The oil simply runs out and is caught and filtered.

✳ **Macerated oils** are actually 'carrier' oils (see pages 24–25) and not pure essential oils. Plant material is gathered and chopped, then added to either sunflower or olive oil. The mix is agitated gently for a while, before being placed in strong sunlight for several days. All of the soluble compounds present in the plant material, including the essential oil, are transferred to the sunflower or olive oil. The mixture is then filtered carefully to remove all the added plant material. What is left is the carrier oil containing the molecules of the essential oil. Plants used for this process are calendula, carrot root and St John's wort (also known as hypericum).

✳ **Solvent extraction** is used to obtain essential oils from plants that do not produce a high yield of essential oils within their oil glands. The flowers are picked and

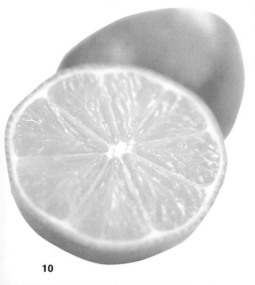

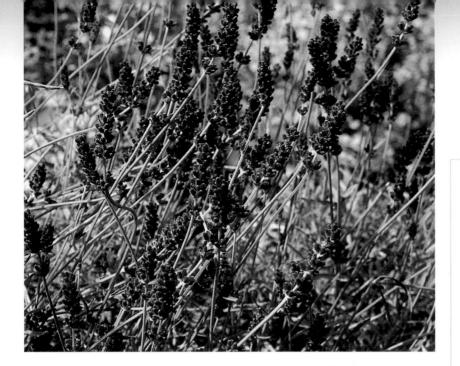

Storing oils

Chemical degradation is the process by which the quality of the essential oil is reduced over a period of time. The three main reasons for the degradation of essential oils are atmospheric oxygen, heat and light. When oxygen is introduced to essential oils, it changes the components within the oil. This process is known as oxidation, and it tends to occur in essential oils rich in terpenes (see page 14), such as lemon and pine. Heat and light also speed up oxidation, so it is important to store essential oils in dark, airtight bottles away from heat and light.

Undiluted essential oils should be used within one year of opening the bottle, and stored in a cool, dark place, preferably in a box. Always buy essential oils in a dark glass bottle – never in a clear glass bottle. If essential oils are stored in the correct manner, they should last up to two years. The exception to this is citrus oils, which should be used within six months of purchase, or one year if kept cool.

immersed in a suitable perfume solvent, which absorbs the smell, colour and wax of the plant. The solvent is then evaporated away to leave a substance known as 'concrete'. The concrete is mixed with alcohol to help filter the waxes. The next process is to distil the alcohol away, which leaves an 'absolute'. This method can be used for rose and jasmine, and the word 'absolute' will appear on the label of the bottled oil. However, because the finished product still contains 2–3 per cent of the solvent, these oils are not pure essential oils.

Caution: Do not confuse rose absolute and rose otto. Rose otto is a pure essential oil that has been steam distilled, and the word 'otto' will appear on the label of the bottle; if it is not there, there is no guarantee that it is a pure rose distilled oil.

Buying oils

Pure-quality essential oils are not easy to find, but synthetic or perfumed oils can cause skin sensitivity. Try to find a reputable mail-order company or retail outlet that not only sells essential oils but can also offer substantial help and advice on their safety and use. Bottles labelled 'Aromatherapy Oil' usually contain essential oils that have been blended in a grapeseed oil. These oils may seem inexpensive, but when you are only receiving 5–10 drops of essential oil in total they are actually very expensive. They will also not have the holistic healing properties of a pure-quality essential oil. The floral waters and natural products mentioned in this book can all be obtained from mail-order and retail outlets that specialize in natural remedies.

History of aromatherapy

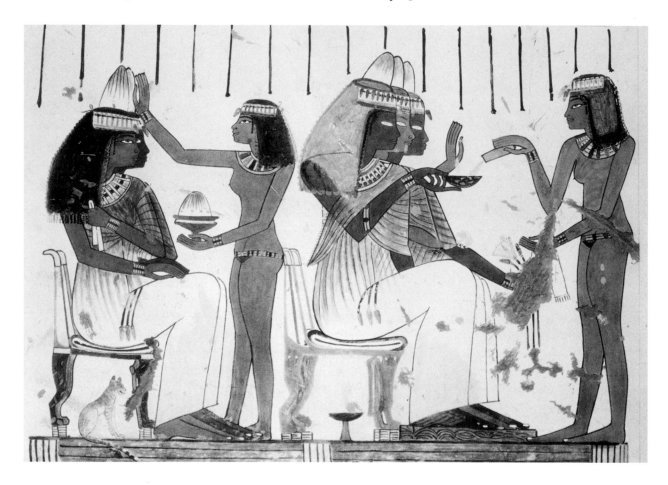

The ancient world

As far back as 4500 BCE, the Egyptians used perfumes. Each Egyptian deity had its own special fragrance, and statues were covered with scented oils. The Egyptians used oils for embalming and forecast that their embalmed bodies would last for 3,000 years.

The ancient Greek physician Hippocrates, known as the 'father of medicine', said that 'the way to health is to have an aromatic bath and scented massage every day'.

The ancient Hindu system of medicine, Ayurveda, incorporated plant extracts and essential oils into its healing potions. In Christianity, according to the Book of Exodus in the Bible, the Lord transmitted to Moses the formula for special anointing oil, which included myrrh, cinnamon, calamus, cassia and olive oil. This holy oil was used to consecrate Moses's brother Aaron, the first high priest of the Israelites.

Above Copy of a wall painting depicting a banqueting scene from the tomb of Nebamun, Thebes, *c.*1400 BCE.

Aromatherapy in Europe

Rose was native to the Orient, and was introduced into Europe by means of the Crusades. To preserve the aroma, they steeped the petals in olive oil. In 14th-century Europe, pine was burned in the street and floors were covered with aromatic plants as a protection against infectious diseases. During the 15th to 17th centuries, several books of herbal remedies, including methods of extracting and using oils, were published throughout Europe. In England, Nicholas Culpeper's famous *Herbal* appeared in 1653.

In the 19th century, essential oils were widely used in medicines. Many aromatic materials filled the pharmacies, which for many centuries remained the main protection against epidemics. Research into essential oils such as cedar, cinnamon, frankincense, juniper, lavender, rosemary, rose and sage continued, and newer oils were developed, such as cajuput, chervil, neroli, valerian and pine. The perfumery and distillation industries thrived in northern Europe, especially at Grasse in France, and flourishing commercial enterprises sprang up.

The term 'aromatherapy' was coined by the French chemist René-Maurice Gattefossé, who grew up around Lyon around the beginning of the 20th century. His research showed that many essential oils were better antiseptics than the synthetics in use at that time. When he applied lavender to serious and gangrenous burns on his arm and head, he found that they healed quickly and left no scarring. He first used the term 'aromatherapie' in articles he wrote, and for the title of his first book, published in 1928.

Aromatherapy today

Modern aromatherapy stems from the work of René-Maurice Gattefossé. Studies have been made throughout the world by laboratory scientists and by practising therapists. Most of this research – somewhat constrained by the dominant scientific ideology – almost exclusively concerns the antiseptic and antibiotic powers of essential oils and their allopathic properties (treating illness by introducing a condition different from the cause of the disease). Research is being carried out in the fields of coronary care, care of the elderly and sleep disorders.

Since the early 1980s, following the work of professors Dodd and Van Toller at Warwick University, UK, a better understanding of the mechanisms of olfaction has opened up new, exciting avenues for research and experimentation in aromatherapy. In retrospect, however, it is clear that the greatest advance made in the development of aromatherapy is the return to genuine oils derived exclusively from one species of plant. Only now are producers of essential oils beginning to manufacture oils according to these requirements.

Below The Paris office of the Societé Française des Produits Aromatiques, France, pictured in 1932.

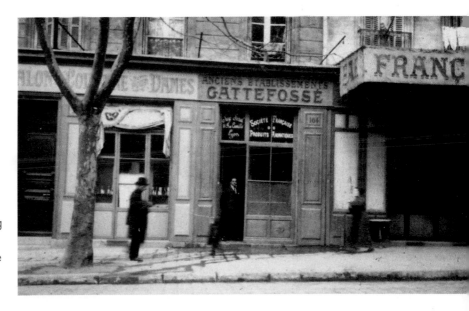

Healing power of oils

Because essential oils are so sweet-smelling, it might be easy to suppose that their value is essentially one of perfume alone. This is a mistake, because these substances are very complex in their molecular structure, and constitute a powerful means by which to promote healing within and around us.

On average, an essential oil contains 100 components. Technology is allowing more of the components within the plants to be identified, and the more we learn about these, the more we are able to understand how aromatherapy works. The main chemical components of essential oils are:

❋ terpenes
❋ alcohols
❋ esters
❋ aldehydes
❋ ketones
❋ phenols

Therapeutic properties

The properties within a living plant that support its very existence are captured in essential oils and used for healing within aromatherapy. Synthetic materials, which may look and smell the same as an essential oil, do not possess these same therapeutic healing qualities. For effective therapeutic use, it is crucial that only pure essential oils are used – that is, natural plant essences, which have been extracted by steam distillation, expression or maceration (see pages 10–11).

There is no point in buying synthetic perfumes, no matter how beautiful their aroma, because reconstituted products or chemical copies of natural essences simply do not work for medicinal purposes. It is the chemical composition of the natural plant that promotes healing within the essential oil.

Adulteration

The world of essential oils is filled with confusion, uncertainty and ignorance concerning the quality of a pure essential oil. Many have been adulterated in some way including diluting, cutting, stretching and ennobling. All these terms mean basically the same thing – the essential oil has been altered from its natural state. It is possible to 'read' the formula of essential oils by means of scientific testing, but this will not show whether the oil is pure or true, because a synthetic perfume will show the same component ratio. What such tests do show is whether the oil has had a substance added or taken away.

Without access to such specialized tests, how is it possible to judge the quality and purity of any oil we may wish to purchase? Sometimes price is the key. It is important to remember that, although poor oil may be bought at a high price, good oil cannot be bought at a low price. Find out from any trader the extent of their knowledge of essential oils with regard to purity, use and safety; try to find a supplier whom you can trust.

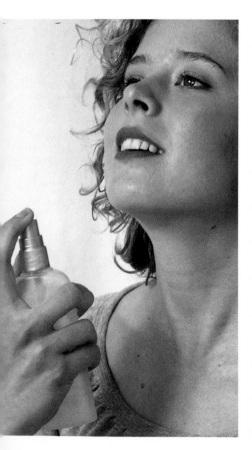

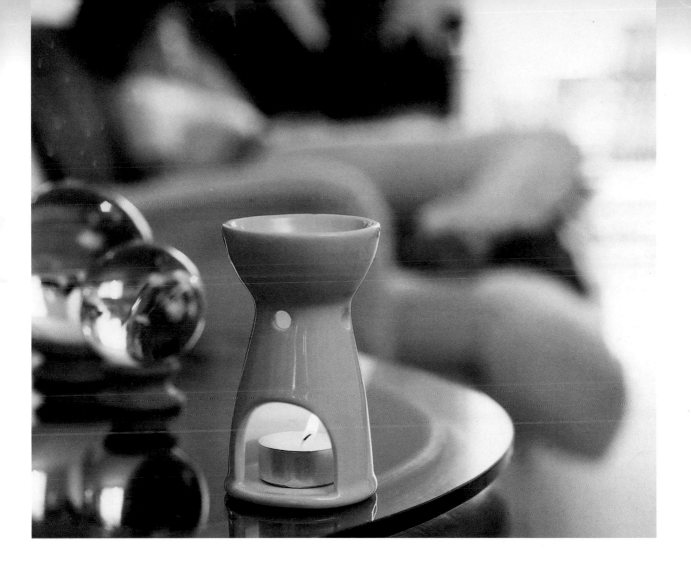

How oils promote well-being

Each essential oil has its own chemical component that has sustained life for the plant. The beneficial effects of these components for the human body can be, among others, sedative, stimulating, pain-relieving, hormone-balancing or diuretic.

There is evidence to show that immunity and resistance to disease is linked to attitudes and behaviour. For many people in today's world, life is a time of chaos, crisis and great opportunity. This creates stress, whether it is constructive or destructive. Studies have shown that depression, as a psychological state, is not sufficient on its own to predict a diminished immune system. However, depression does play a role, in that the more severe the depression, the more likely it is that a decreased measure of immune response will be found.

Aromatherapy addresses itself to the physical, mental and spiritual aspects of those who need care. It views health as a positive state, not as the absence of disease. It emphasizes the uniqueness of the individual and the importance of tailoring treatments to meet each person's need. When you smell and enjoy the aroma of the essential oil you are using, tiny molecules penetrate the body via the nose and send tiny chemical messages to the brain to uplift the mind and spirit.

How the body absorbs essential oils

Cross-section of the olfactory system

limbic system
(sensory/emotional/hormonal integration)

septum

olfactory bulb

olfactory cilia hair

odour molecule

hypothalamus

amygdala

olfactory tract

olfactory cortex

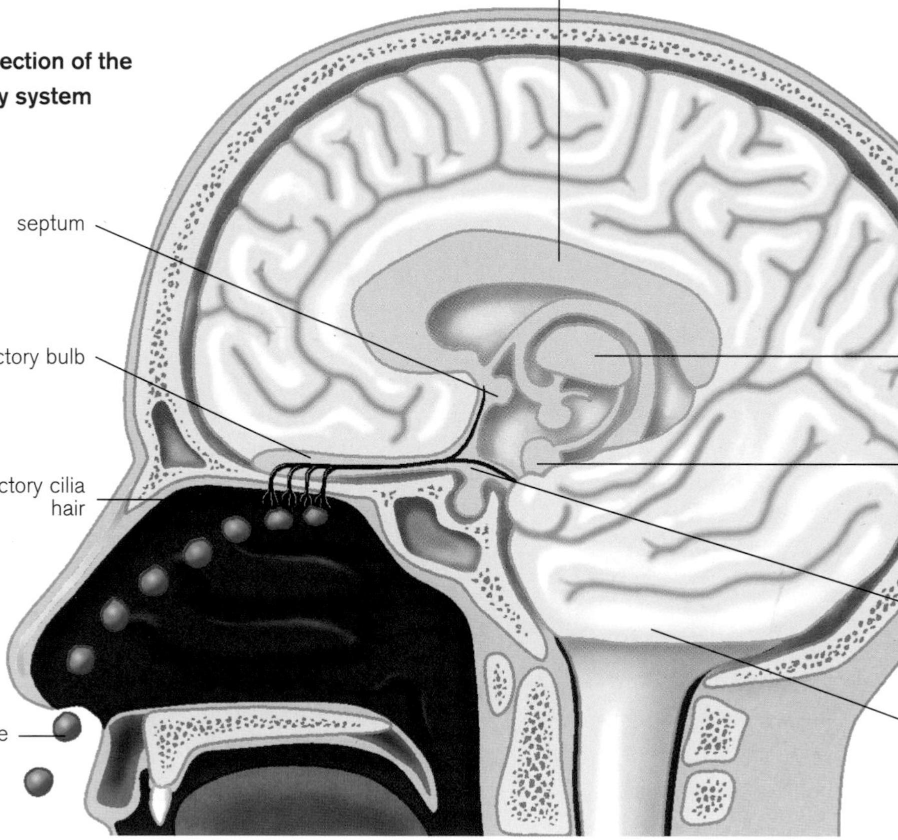

The olfactory system

Smell (olfaction) has always been one of the most important human senses. It is used to detect the presence of vital aspects concerning basic survival, such as food, enemies and the opposite sex.

When essential oils are inhaled, the tiny molecules are taken directly to the roof of the nose, where the receptor cells of the olfactory system are situated. Each receptor cell protrudes thin hairs, which are called cilia. The cilia hairs register and transmit the information about the aromas, via the olfactory bulb, to the centre of the brain. From here,

electrochemical messages are sent to the parts of the brain associated with smell. These trigger the release of neurochemicals, which may be sedative, relaxing, stimulating or euphoric in effect. Aromatic molecules also travel down the nasal passages to the lungs where they are diffused into the bloodstream via the lungs.

The skin

When essential oils are applied externally to the skin, the oils are absorbed into the bloodstream by passing through the sweat glands and hair follicles. The hair follicles contain sebum, an oily liquid that aids the absorption of the essential oil. From here, the oils diffuse into the bloodstream and are taken by the lymph and interstitial fluid (a liquid surrounding all body cells) to other parts of the body.

The essential oils are absorbed at varying rates into the body. 'Top note' essential oils (see pages 22–23) will enter the body more quickly, because they have tiny molecules that reach the systemic circulation within half an hour of application. The slowest essential oils to reach the bloodstream are the 'base notes' (see page 23), because they have a much heavier and larger molecule structure. A classic test of the skin's ability to absorb substances is to rub a clove of garlic onto the soles of the feet; the odour will be detected on the breath within an hour.

Cross-section of the skin

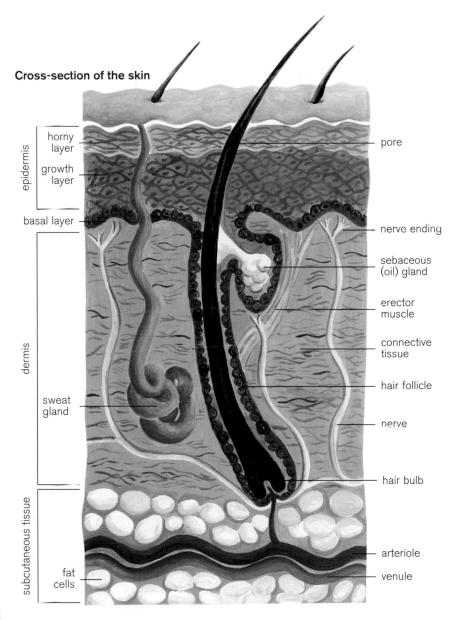

epidermis
- horny layer
- growth layer

basal layer

dermis

subcutaneous tissue

- sweat gland
- fat cells

- pore
- nerve ending
- sebaceous (oil) gland
- erector muscle
- connective tissue
- hair follicle
- nerve
- hair bulb
- arteriole
- venule

Handy hint

A factor that helps the essential oils to penetrate the skin quickly is body warmth. Have a warm bath or use friction massage on the area where you want to apply the essential oils.

Caution: When the skin is damaged or diseased, the rate of absorption is greatly increased. This means that the risk of a skin reaction increases. Essential oils should always be applied with caution to damaged skin.

Methods of use

The main ways of using essential oils are massage, bathing, inhalation and vaporizing. Other methods also used include taking a sauna and applying compresses. You may wish to try some or all of the following methods before deciding which is the best for you. Your choice of method may also depend on your reason for using a particular oil or blend of oils.

Massage

Massage is an important part of an aromatherapy treatment. Touching is a very sensuous and comforting part of human interaction. When touching takes the form of a skilled but sensitive massage, it relaxes and revitalizes an ailing or tired body. It is a way of communicating reassurance and a sense of self-worth. When you combine essential oils with massage, you enter a world of healing enhanced with the touch of healing hands and the aroma of healing fragrance. This in itself will help lift depression and go towards healing the body. Massage is one of the most effective ways of using essential oils.

Blending massage oils

For massage, the essential oils are always blended in vegetable-based carrier oils (see pages 24–25). Never put neat essential oils onto the skin. Remember to choose essential oils that you like the smell of.

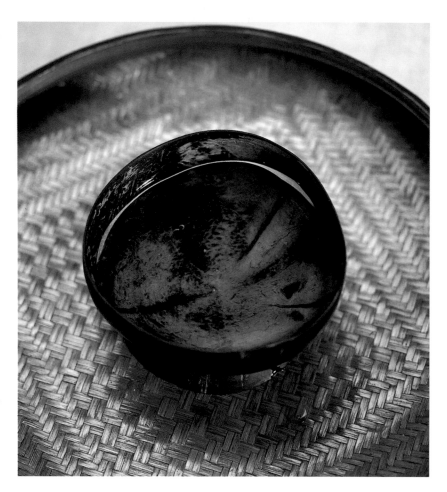

✴ For adults, add up to 6 drops of essential oil to 15ml (½fl oz) vegetable carrier oil. Use either a single oil or one of the synergistic blends (see page 22, and those recommended throughout the book) that will benefit a particular condition you want to treat.

✴ To make a suitable massage oil for children under 12 years old, add 2 drops of essential oil to 20ml (¾fl oz) vegetable carrier oil.

✴ For babies under 3 years old, add 1 drop of essential oil to 50ml (2fl oz) organic sunflower oil. Organic sunflower oil is best, because other vegetable carriers generally come from nuts or seeds, which can be allergenic to young children and babies.

Bathing

Bathing is another effective way of using essential oils. They are normally used in a relaxing bath, but can also be used while showering, or in a hand or foot bath.

Taking a bath
❋ Run a warm bath; add up to 4–6 drops of your favourite essential oil, either a single essential oil or a synergistic blend (see pages 22–23).

❋ If you have dry or sensitive skin, add the synergistic blend to 10ml (⅙fl oz) of unscented foam or milk base (obtainable from all good suppliers of aromatherapy products), which will help disperse the essential oil.

❋ Allow yourself to soak in the bath for at least 10 minutes, giving time for the essential oils to penetrate the body and relax and soothe you.

Bathing babies and children
❋ For babies under 3 years old, mix 1 drop of essential oil with 10ml (⅙fl oz) unscented bath milk base. This will disperse the oil and not leave any globules of the oil lying on top of the bath, which can cause irritation on young, sensitive skin.

❋ For children under 12 years old, run a full bath and mix in 2 drops of essential oil to 10ml (⅙fl oz) unscented bath milk base.

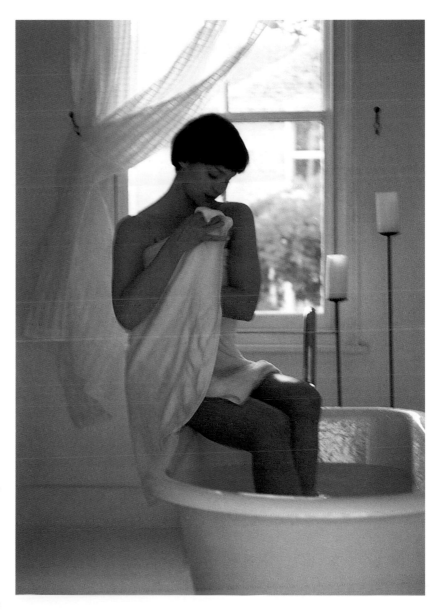

Caution: Avoid splashing bathwater in the eyes.

Taking a shower
If you prefer to take a shower rather than have a bath, add 6 drops of essential oils or synergistic blend to 50ml (2fl oz) of unscented shower gel, and use as normal.

Do not add essential oils to commercially scented shower or bath preparations, because this could cause a sensitizing reaction to the skin. You can buy unscented bath preparations from any good supplier of aromatherapy products.

Using a hand or foot bath

Blend 5 drops of essential oil to 10ml (⅙fl oz) unscented bath milk base, and add to a bowl of warm water or a spa. Soak the hands or feet for 10–20 minutes.

Using oils in a sauna

Mix 2 drops of essential oils with 600ml (1 pint) of water and throw it onto the heat source in the usual way. Do not use any more than 2 drops of essential oil, since some of the oils (especially eucalyptus and peppermint) can make your eyes water if the proportions used are too strong.

Caution: Do not use any of the citrus oils in a sauna if you are going straight onto a sunbed. Citrus oils are phototoxic, which means they will cause the skin to blister or burn.

Steam inhalation

A simple way of inhaling oils is to put 1–2 drops of neat essential oil onto a handkerchief or tissue and inhale when required.

Steam inhalation, in which steam vapours are breathed in through the nose, is very useful for relieving colds, headaches, congestion and catarrh. For a safe and effective steam inhalation, follow these instructions:

✳ Place 600ml to 1 litre (1–2 pints) of warm water into a bowl.

✳ Add 2–6 drops of essential oils (use either a single oil or a synergistic blend).

✳ Put a towel over your head and over the bowl, close your eyes and inhale the vapours deeply through your nose for about one minute.

✳ Do not put your face too close to the steam, as this could burn your skin.

✳ Repeat the inhalation several times a day if required.

If you prefer, you can use essential oils with a facial steamer instead of a bowl. You should add 2–6 drops of essential oils and inhale for about one minute.

Caution: Do not use the inhalation method or dab neat essential oils onto the skin or clothes of young children or babies. The oils are too strong and can cause a serious reaction.

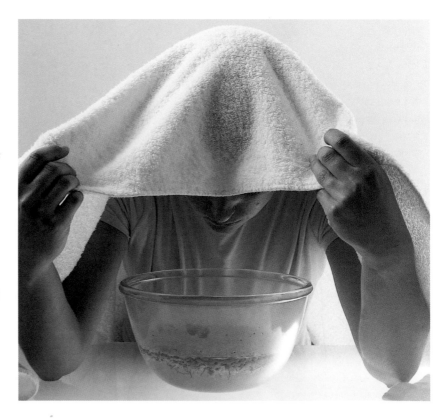

Vaporizing

There are several ways of vaporizing essential oils to create a perfumed atmosphere in a room.

Essential-oil burners

These generally consist of a ceramic or metal pot with a small reservoir or container at the top. The small reservoir is for holding water; this helps stop the pot from overheating. A nightlight candle is lit and placed inside the burner. Sprinkle up to 10 drops of essential oil into the water. The heat from the flame vaporizes the aroma from the essential oils in the air. Do not place carrier oil into the reservoir because the oil will heat up and cause a serious burn if spilt.

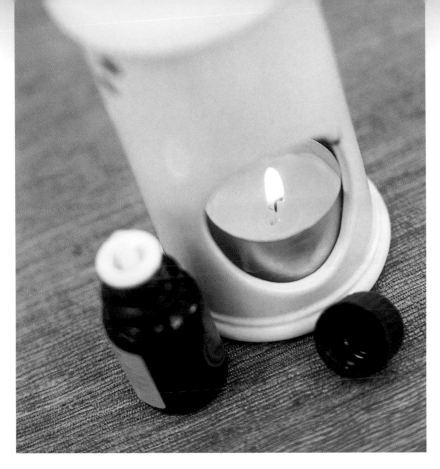

Diffusers

These are electric units especially designed for safety and use with essential oils. Up to 12 drops of essential oils may be added to these diffusers, and when plugged in and working they do not overheat.

If you want to provide fragrance in a room for young children or elderly people, always use a diffuser rather than a ceramic or metal pot.

Humidifiers

A saucer of water with up to 12 drops of essential oils placed on top of a radiator will act both as a vaporizer and humidifier.

Room sprays

Fill a plant spray bottle with 300ml (10fl oz) warm water and add up to 10 drops of single essential oil or a synergistic blend (see pages 22–23). Shake before use.

Perfume

Blend a carrier oil with a synergistic blend (as directed for the particular ailment or room; see pages 54–115). Pour the blend into a bottle and use it as you would a normal perfume.

Using compresses

A compress is a pack of cloth or gauze pad, usually dampened with hot or cold water, that is pressed firmly against a part of the body to relieve discomfort. As it is only applied to a small area or part of the body, a stronger blend can be used.

For adults, up to 10 drops of essential oil can be blended with 20ml (¾fl oz) of a vegetable carrier oil for the massage.

✳ Gently massage the part of the body that is causing discomfort or pain with the massage mixture.

✳ Place a warm or cold compress on the area massaged, and leave for 30 minutes. Use a warm compress for aches and pains, and a cold compress for inflammation, temperature and sprains.

Blending essential oils

Within the perfume industry, the person responsible for creating perfumes is known as the 'nose'. This very important 'perfumer' must know and work with several thousand different products and scents in order to create a single perfume. After working with a succession of different combinations, the perfumer attempts to create a well-balanced and pleasant fragrance.

Most people cannot expect to be trained 'noses', but are aware of aromas that they like and enjoy. The following section helps to make blending different essential oils together both easy and understandable.

Synergistic blends

When essential oils are blended together, they can actually work better than they would if used separately; for example, when lavender is mixed with camomile, the anti-inflammatory action of the camomile is enhanced. When the blended oils are working harmoniously together in this way, the combination is called a 'synergy'. To create a good synergy, you must take into account not only the symptom to be treated but also the underlying cause of the disorder.

Guidelines on synergistic blends for specific conditions and situations are provided throughout the rest of

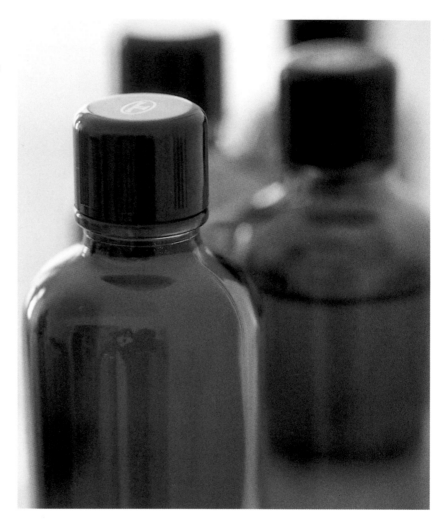

this book. The essential oils chosen will benefit the condition that the oils need to treat. Each person's condition is unique, and you will need to find out which essential oil and blends work best for you. Use the synergistic blend as a guideline for your blending, but also smell and try the other essential oils quoted in the

'Other useful essential oils' section for each ailment, because you may find that they suit you better.

The essential oils are very powerful, so please respect the indicated amounts. If the blend states 2 drops of peppermint, do not be tempted to add an extra 3–4 drops, thinking that it will work better; it will

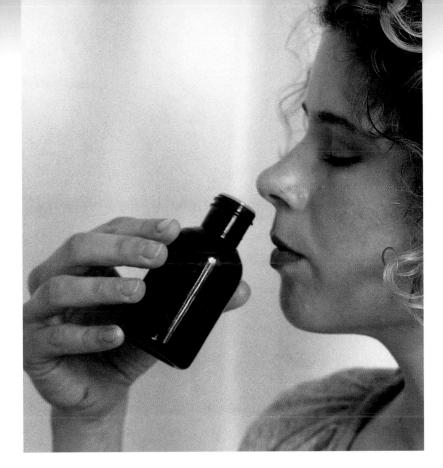

are often warm, round, soft and mellow. Middle notes typically form the bulk of the blend.

✳ **Base notes** are the fixatives; they deepen your blend and draw it into the skin, giving it roots and permanence. When smelled from the bottle, base notes seem rather faint, but when applied to the skin they react strongly and release their power.

Blending top, middle and base notes

Another way of blending essential oils is by using the top, middle and base notes of the essential oils. See the Directory of essential oils (pages 116–123) to identify whether an oil is a top, middle or base note.

To make a blend that is balanced, choose essential oils that you enjoy the aroma of. Out of the group of oils you like, choose one oil that is a top note, one a middle note and one a base note. Blend these as 2 drops of top, 3 drops of middle and 1 drop of base in 15ml (½fl oz) of carrier oil. This way the all-round perfume of the blend will have a balanced smell, and no one oil will dominate the others.

not, and may only serve to irritate the skin. You may wish to use less than the indicated amounts, however, since sometimes a more diluted blend can be just as effective.

Top, middle and base notes

When you open an essential-oil bottle, the first smell that hits you consists of 'top note' molecules. After a few seconds, the heavier molecules start to evaporate and you begin to smell the whole aroma of the essential oil, including the 'middle notes' and the 'base notes'. This is why when smelling the perfume of

the oil your first reaction may be positive but after a while you change your mind. It is the heavier molecules escaping the bottle at a later stage that you are rejecting. It is best to pour a little of the oil onto a tissue or testing strip, as this will give you the full aroma when you smell it.

✳ **Top notes** hit you first. They do not last long, but they are very important because they give the first impression of the blend. They are sharp, penetrating, volatile, extreme and either cold or hot, but never warm.

✳ **Middle notes** give body to your blends; they smooth the sharp edges and round the angles. They

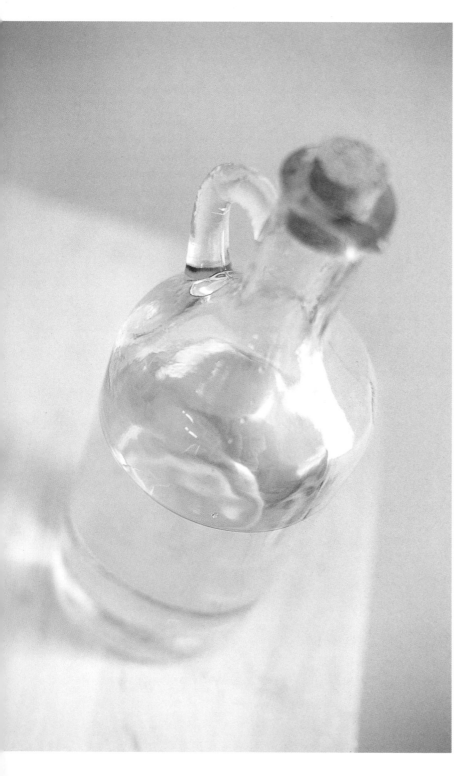

Carrier oils

The essential oils are very powerful, concentrated substances that should never be applied directly onto the skin because an adverse reaction could occur. A 'carrier' oil is an odourless vegetable oil, such as sunflower oil, that is used as a base medium to which are added a few drops of essential oil before use. Essential oils are very rarely used without being diluted either in water or in a carrier oil. Your skin will benefit if you use cold-pressed vegetable oils as a carrier, because these are rich in vitamins B and E.

The following are among the most common carrier oils (see also the Directory of carrier oils on pages 124–125), and they can be used with or without essential oils for body massage. They are generally pale in colour, not too thick and have very little smell.

✳ sweet almond
✳ apricot kernel
✳ grapeseed
✳ peach kernel
✳ sunflower

Heavy viscous carrier oils

Certain vegetable oils tend to be more viscous and heavier than basic carrier oils, and can be rather expensive. Because of the richness of these oils, they are considered too heavy to use on their own. Therefore, up to 25 per cent of one of the following more viscous oils (see also pages 124–125) can be added to the basic carrier oils. This will give an enriched carrier for different skin complaints, making this an ideal individual blend.

* avocado
* evening primrose
* jojoba
* rose hip
* wheatgerm (may cause an allergic reaction in some people)
* neem seed

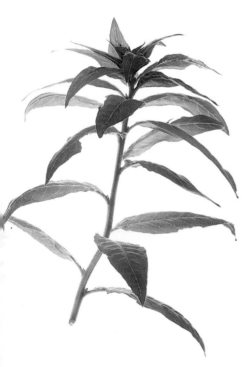

Evening primrose
Oenetheris biennis

Cold-pressed vegetable oils

In the 'cold' pressing process, excessive heat is avoided in order to minimize changes to the natural characteristics of the oil. Traditionally, there are two methods of cold pressing. In one, the raw material (seeds, nuts or kernels) is simply pressed with a hydraulic press and the oil is squeezed out. This process is only used for soft oily seeds and plant material, such as olive, sesame and sunflower.

Harder nuts or seeds require more force. The nuts or seeds are placed in a horizontal press with an enormous 'screw'. As this turns, the oil is squeezed out and drips into a trough below. The first oil to be collected is known as 'virgin-pressed' (olive oil is commercially available in virgin and second pressings). Natural heat is generated as the pressure increases to force out more oil, but careful watch is kept to see that it does not reach 70–80°C (160–180°F). If it reaches a higher temperature than this, the oil cannot be classed as cold-pressed. After pressing, the oil is filtered in successive cotton cloths and finally

through a paper filter. The oil obtained is usually clear (avocado is an exception as it is usually cloudy, especially in cold conditions) with its taste and nutritional properties intact.

Macerated oils

Macerated carrier oils have additional properties because of the way in which they are produced (see page 10). Use up to 25 per cent macerated oil when blending with a basic carrier oil.

Blending with carrier oils

The carrier oils are nourishing, healing and soothing to the skin. When blending for certain ailments and conditions, consult the Directory of carrier oils (see pages 124–125) and mix a selection of these with your essential oils. You will soon see a difference in the condition of your skin. The following blends are recommended.

* Mature skin: apricot kernel, carrot and rose hip.
* Dry skin: sweet almond, avocado and wheatgerm.
* Oily skin: jojoba and hypericum.

Massage

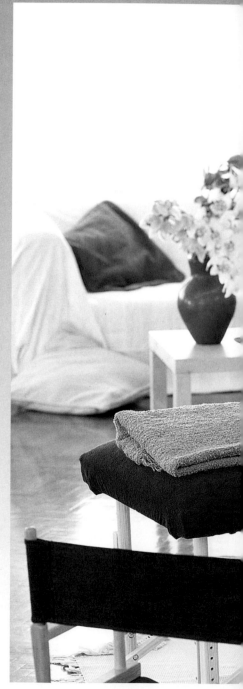

Humans are very sensitive, tactile creatures. When we hurt ourselves, we rub the area to make it better and ease the pain. We comfort those who are upset with a hug. In this respect, stroking and caressing may be just as important to our health as food and cleanliness. Massage is an advanced and conscious form of the instinctive and innate ability to offer healing through the hands.

Skilled massage relaxes and revitalizes an ailing or tired body, and also communicates warmth, reassurance and a sense of self-worth. In aromatherapy, the relaxing effects of massage combined with the beneficial properties of essential oils can promote well-being of body, mind and spirit.

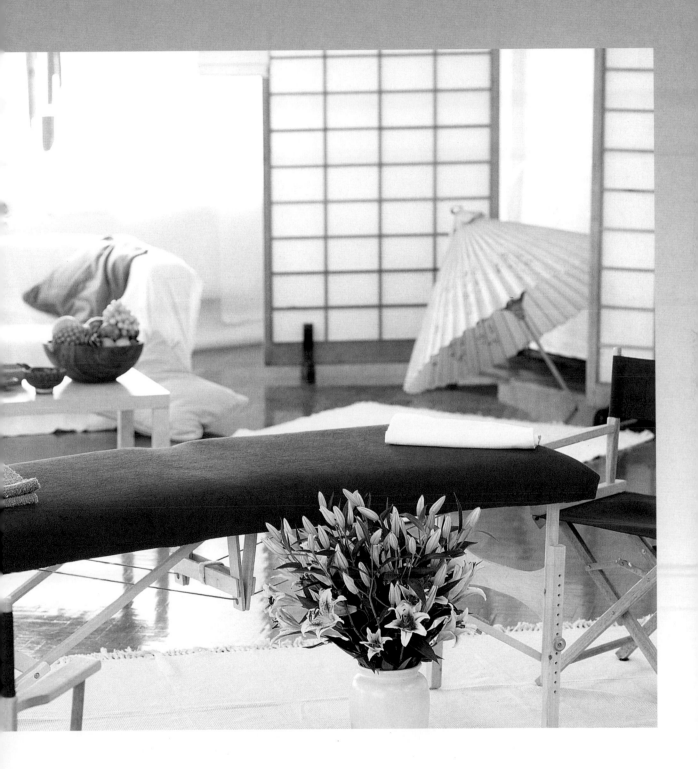

Preparation

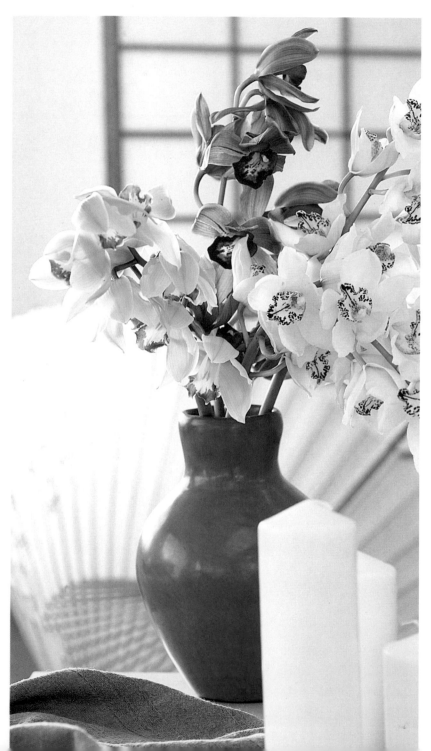

In order for massage to be truly beneficial, the masseur, or 'giver', and the 'receiver' both need to be in the right mood. If the giver has had a difficult day, sometimes the resultant stress can be communicated to the receiver. The receiver, to benefit fully from massage, must learn to receive massage passively. If they constantly chatter and fidget, it is difficult for them to receive the benefits of the massage. So first make sure that you are both feeling relaxed and positive.

The massage area

Choose a peaceful room with a relaxing ambience. The surroundings should be warm and inviting. Harsh colours, untidy clutter and noise will make a room feel irritating and claustrophobic, and will build a barrier preventing a healing atmosphere from developing. Neutral colours or pastel shades are conducive to relaxation and healing. To create a restful room, soft light, fresh flowers and a bowl of fruit or crystals will nurture all the senses. Lift the spirit of the room with relaxation music, playing at a low volume so that it is only in the background.

If you do not have a massage couch or a sturdy wooden table, you will have to work at floor level. This is not always a good idea for the masseur, because it can hurt the knees and back. For the receiver it is

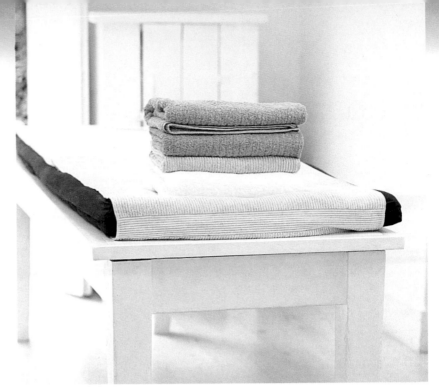

better, however, since it is easier for the masseur to apply beneficial pressure using their own bodyweight. Never massage a person on a bed, because the surface is too soft and you will not be able to apply pressure when working.

You will need a few blankets, or perhaps a folded duvet covered with towels, to provide the necessary comfortable padding under the receiver. When using towels, a bath sheet is the best size to use, since you want to make sure that the receiver does not catch cold or feel chilled during the massage. When massaging, only expose the area being massaged and keep the rest of the body covered. A professional therapist never leaves a body completely uncovered, not only for reasons of warmth and modesty but also because it can make a person feel vulnerable.

Preparing oils

Prepare a synergistic blend of essential oils – choose a blend that is appropriate to the condition or emotional state of the receiver (see pages 54–101). You will need about 20ml (¾fl oz) to complete a full body massage. If you intend to massage only one part of the body – the face, back or feet, for example – then no more than 10ml (⅙fl oz) of oil are needed. Never pour the oil directly

onto the body. Ensure that your hands are warm, and pour a small amount into the palm of your hand. Then rub your hands together before applying to the receiver's body.

Aims and benefits of massage:
* To increase or decrease the energy level of the body.
* To increase circulation of lymphatic fluids in order to increase the release of toxins.
* To break down waste deposits in tired or aching muscles.
* To tone underworked or weak muscles.
* To help with suppressed feelings.
* To promote good posture.

Caution: Never massage a person who has any of the following conditions without seeking medical advice:

* a fever or an infection
* recent surgery or a fracture
* high or low blood pressure
* diabetes
* a serious condition such as heart disease or cancer
* pregnancy
* varicose veins
* epilepsy
* swollen joints associated with arthritis and rheumatic conditions

Basic techniques

The massage sequence described on pages 34–47 is a modified version of a professional aromatherapy massage. It is based on four basic massage movements.

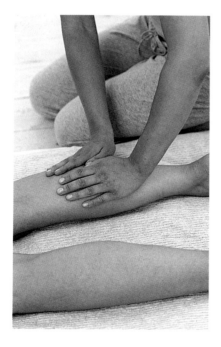

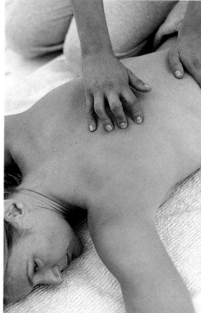

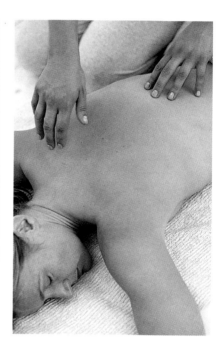

Effleurage: a form of long, stroking movement, using the whole surface of the hand.

Friction: where pressure is applied with the ball of the thumb or fingers, and then moved in small circles over a particular area.

Feathering: short, light, fingertip stroking; the fingers move gently behind each other in a continuous movement, moving off after stroking around 5cm (2in).

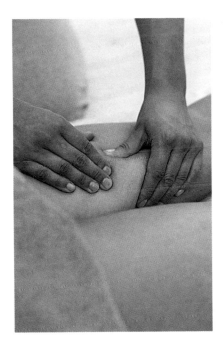

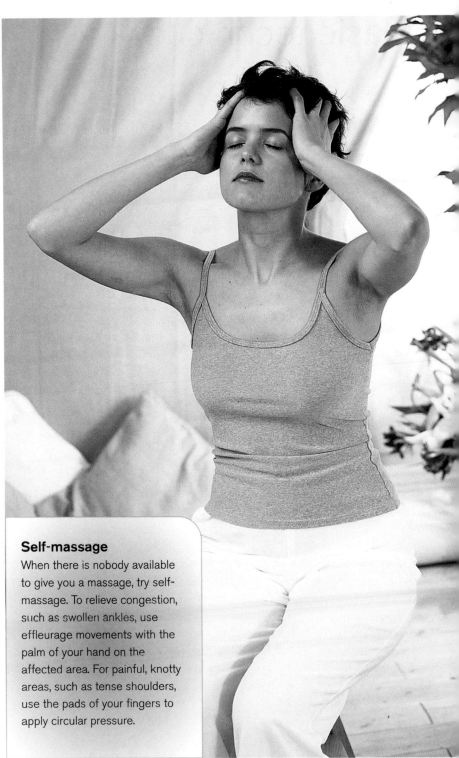

Kneading: a movement that involves the hands working together, gently picking up and squeezing a fleshy part of muscle (a similar action to kneading bread dough).

(Percussion, which is a form of hacking, pounding or cupping, is rarely used in aromatherapy massage. These types of movements are more commonly used in sports or remedial massage.)

Self-massage

When there is nobody available to give you a massage, try self-massage. To relieve congestion, such as swollen ankles, use effleurage movements with the palm of your hand on the affected area. For painful, knotty areas, such as tense shoulders, use the pads of your fingers to apply circular pressure.

Watchpoints

It is important to remember all the following points when massaging.

✳ Never pour the oil directly onto the body of the receiver. Ensure that your hands are warm, pour a small amount into the palm of your hand, and then rub your hands together before applying to the receiver's body.

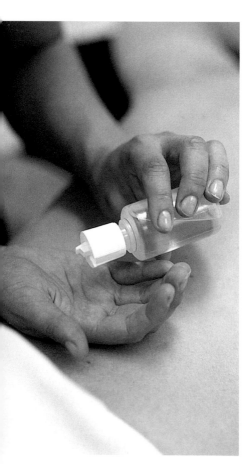

✳ The pressure that is used for aromatherapy massage is firm but with light strokes. You need to feel the muscle under your hands, and the receiver does not want to feel battered or tickled.

✳ When massaging the body, try to keep in contact with the receiver's body throughout the massage, even when you need to apply more oil. The massage should feel like one continuous, flowing movement. To break contact mid-flow will feel disconcerting to the receiver.

✳ Never apply heavy pressure to the spine and bony areas of the body, such as knees and collarbone.

✳ Be firm over large areas of muscle, such as either side of the spine or the buttocks.

✳ Movements in general for aromatherapy massage are slow, deep and calming. These movements tend to relax or stimulate according to the state of the receiver. Receiving an aromatherapy massage has a balancing effect on the body and the mind.

✳ When giving a massage, try to work with the whole of your body and not just your hands and arms. For instance, when applying the long, smooth strokes on the back of the legs, lean into the movement, using your bodyweight rather than just your arm and shoulder muscles. The more relaxed and fluid your own movements, the more relaxed and at ease the receiver will become.

✳ The key to working with the whole of your body is to become aware of your own breathing. Use deep, slow breathing techniques when massaging and this will convey a feeling of relaxation to the receiver.

✳ The sensitivity combined with the joy of giving will make your massage one to be remembered. You do not need to be a professional masseur to give a rewarding massage. The goodwill that goes with touch makes all the difference to its effect.

The massage sequence

Now you should be ready to perform the full body massage sequence (see pages 34–47), starting with the back and finishing off with the face and scalp.

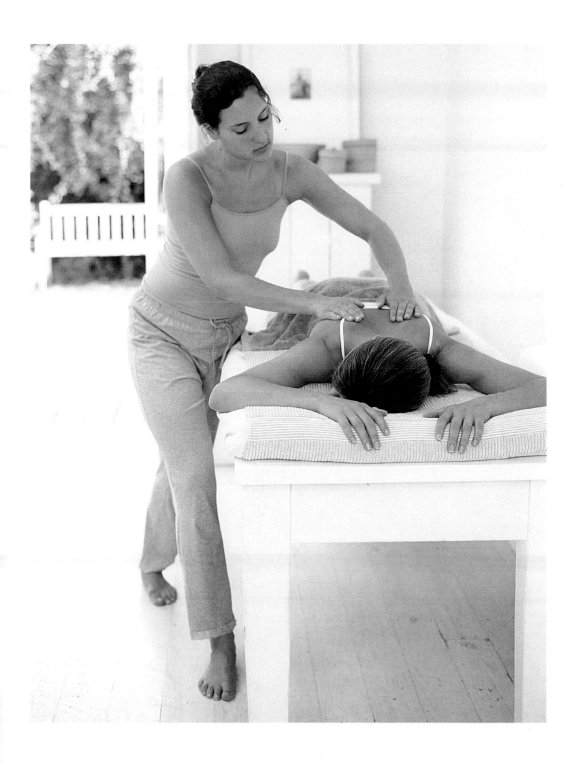

Full body massage sequence

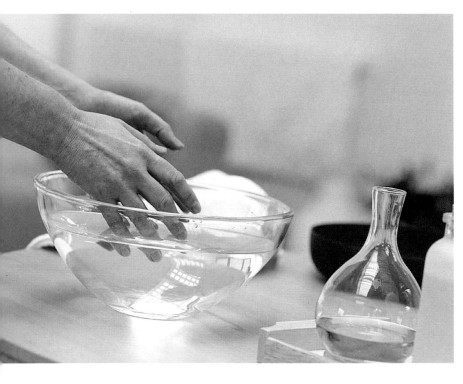

thus enabling you to lean into the strokes. If you are working on the floor, kneel with your knees placed slightly apart.

✳ Before oiling your hands, place them gently onto the top and bottom of the receiver's back. Now ask them to breathe deeply, so that you are able to follow their lead, and breathe together for a few seconds. This will calm you both and will enable the receiver to relax and become accustomed to your touch.

✳ Warm and oil your hands. Pull the towel down to expose half the buttock crease. Apply the oil over the whole of the back, using firm, upward, continuous effleurage movements. Repeat each of the following movements four times.

Back

Preparation

✳ Position the receiver on their front. The head should be to one side, and arms relaxed at the side of the body. Some people feel more comfortable with a rolled-up towel or pillow under their ankles (see right). This takes pressure off their lower back.

✳ Cover your partner from neck to foot with two bath sheets. If you are using a massage table, stand with your feet slightly apart so that you are able to bend at the knees,

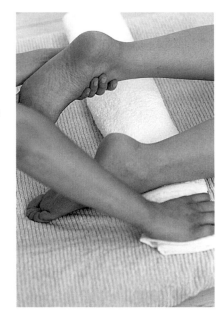

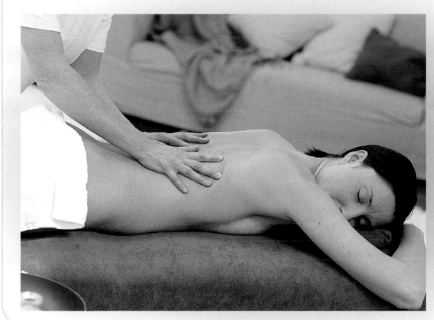

Lymphatic massage

This is an effective massage for improving lymph drainage, that has been developed for the treatment of oedema (fluid retention).

Effleurage the body slowly with the whole of the hand, using very light pressure. The weight of the hand exerts sufficient pressure to move the lymph through the superficial vessels. The direction of the stroke is always towards the nearest lymph nodes.

The movements

1 Beginning at the base of the back, place your hands on either side of the spine, with your fingers fairly close together but relaxed and pointing towards the head. Effleurage your hands up the back on either side of the spine, leaning into the stroke until you reach the neck. Fan out your hands firmly across the shoulders, then glide them down the side of the body with fingers almost touching the table or floor. When you reach the base of the spine and buttock area, pull up gently towards the spine and return smoothly to the starting position.

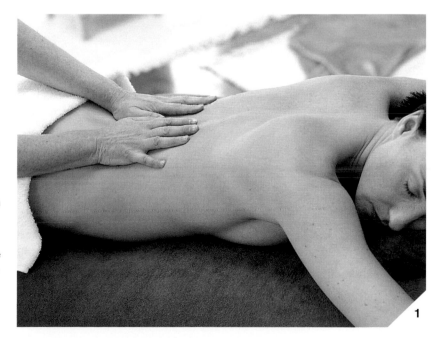

1

2 Starting with your hands on the lower back, as before, effleurage firmly upwards, and when you reach the shoulders, place one hand over the other. With fingers pointing towards the head, give firm effleurage in a figure of eight over each shoulder blade.

3 Open the hands and rest the fingertips over each of the shoulders. With the pad of your thumbs, use deep circle friction between the shoulder blades. You may come across areas of small nodules under the skin, which are caused by bunched-up muscle fibres and an accumulation of waste products. Continue working in this area until you have soothed away any tension you may find. Sometimes the receiver will experience 'therapeutic pain', a dull sensation that will elicit a groan of relief. If it is a shriek of pain, this may mean that the muscle has contracted even harder to protect itself; if this happens, release your pressure immediately.

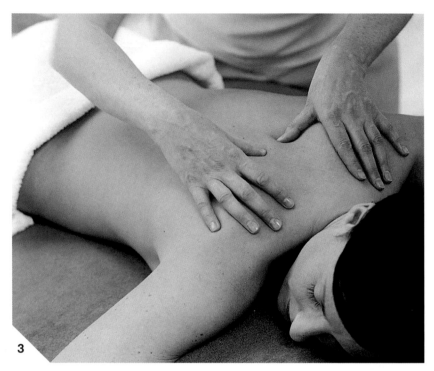

3

4 Release your fingers from the receiver's shoulders, and gently effleurage down the side of the body to the base of the back, where you should begin the back effleurage, as in movement 1.

5 When you reach the base of the spine, position your thumbs at waist level either side of the spinal column. Relax the fingers on either side of

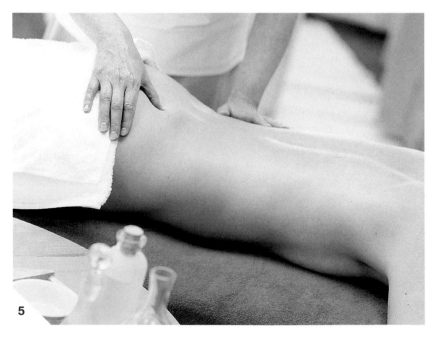

5

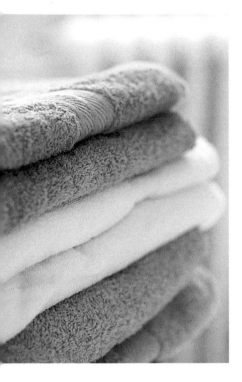

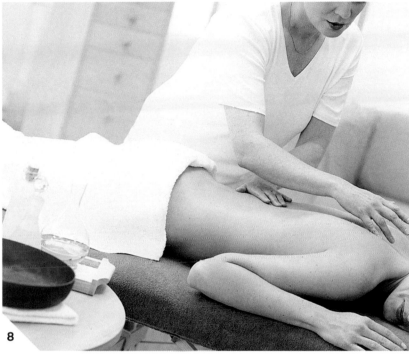

8

the waist, and with the pad of your thumb use deep friction circles, 2.5cm (1in) in diameter, travelling out to the side of the body down towards the table or floor. Draw your fingers back up to the base of the spine and place your thumb each side of the spinal column, 2.5cm (1in) lower down from the previous position. Continue the deep circle friction movement over the lower back and buttock area and down towards the side. Continue with four or five lines covering the whole of the waist, lower back and buttock area.

6 Position both hands, using the flat of the hand, at the waist and lower back. Fan the fingers towards each side of the body, leaving your thumbs pointing towards the head. Apply pressure to the whole palm of the hand, and glide over the waist and buttock area towards the side. Let the hand and fingers relax on the bed, open the hand and bring back to the waist and lower back to repeat the movement.

7 Effleurage the whole of the back, as in movement 1.

8 To finish the back massage, after repeating the effleurage return to the base of the neck and, using short 2.5cm (1in) light feather strokes with your fingertips, gently come down the spine and off at the base of the back.

9 Cover the whole of the back with the towel to keep the receiver warm.

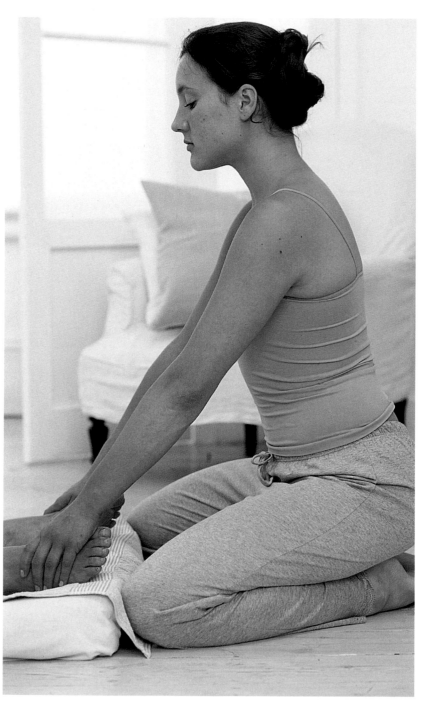

Legs and feet

Back of the leg

Apply oil to your hands and massage oil onto both legs. Place the towel over the right leg to keep it warm. Repeat each of the following movements four times.

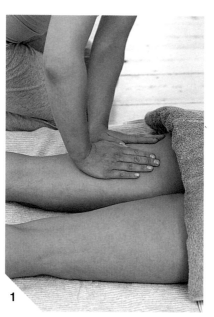

1

1 Working on the left leg, start at the feet. Relax both hands over the base of the leg, and, moving both hands together, effleurage firmly up the leg from the ankle, lightly over the back of the knee, and towards the top of the leg. Keeping contact with the leg, relax the hands and gently slide back down either side of the leg to the feet, to start the movement again.

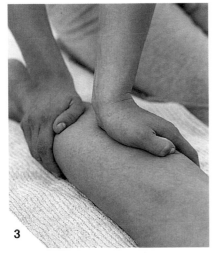

3

2 Place your fingers under the left foot, and lift the foot upright. Support the foot with one hand and effleurage from the ankle to the knee, pressing firmly with the whole palm of the hand. Finish the movement at the ankle, laying the leg gently down.

3 Complete the left leg massage by effleuraging the whole leg, as in movement 1.

4 Cover the left leg to keep it warm, and repeat the above sequence on the right leg.

Front of the leg

Position the receiver on their back, with a cushion or rolled-up towel under the knees to prevent any strain in the lower region of the back. Apply oil to your hands and massage the oil onto both legs, including the feet. Place the towel over the right leg to keep it warm. Repeat each of the following movements four times.

1 Place the palms of your hands, crossed, with fingers relaxed, over each side of the receiver's left foot. Effleurage up the whole of the leg. When you reach the top of the leg, fan your hands and glide gently back down each side of the leg towards the foot.

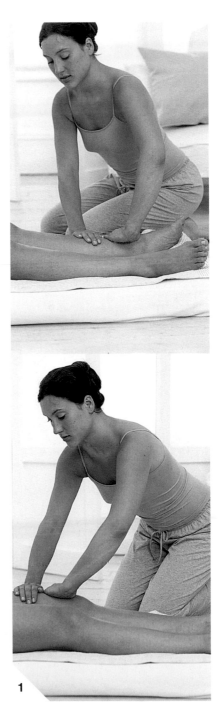

1

2 Glide up to the knee, and place your left hand on the inside of the thigh under the knee. Using diagonal effleurage, with alternate hands lift the inside thigh and stroke out. Start at the knee and finish at the top of the leg.

3 Place your left hand below the kneecap, and with the palm of your right hand, effleurage the outer thigh. Use strong sweeping strokes over the whole of the outer thigh.

4 Complete the massage by repeating movement 1. Cover the left leg to keep it warm, and repeat the above sequence on the right leg.

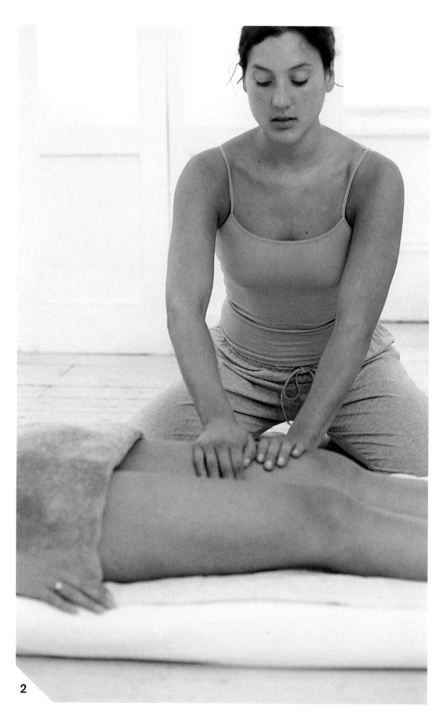

2

Foot

Cover the right leg and foot to keep them warm. Repeat each of the following movements four times.

1 Massage and circle around the left ankle with your fingertips.

2 Slide towards the toes and, with light-friction thumb circles, massage between the small bones on the foot towards the ankle.

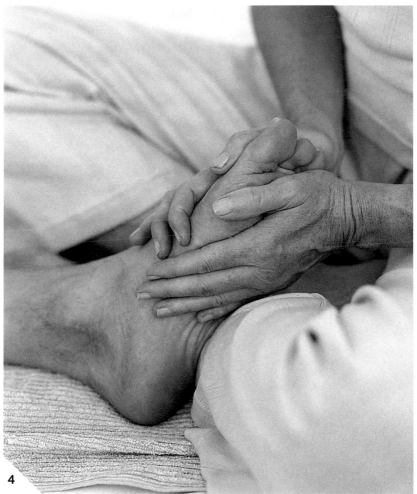

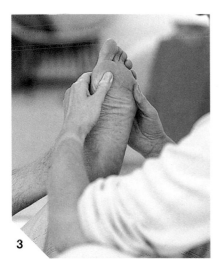

3

4

3 Hold the foot with both hands, with the fingers over the top of the foot and thumbs on the base of the foot, and do a scissor movement with both your thumbs up behind the base of the foot.

4 To complete the left foot massage, gently sandwich the foot between your hand and slide slowly up the foot, moving off at the toe tips.

5 Cover the left leg, remembering to keep the foot warm, and repeat the above sequence on the right foot.

Arms

Apply oil to your hands and massage oil onto the whole of the left hand and arm. Repeat each of the following movements four times.

1 With your left hand, hold the receiver's left hand. With your right hand, using the flat palm, effleurage from the wrist along the whole of the left arm, up to the top of the shoulder. Gently relax the fingers and come back to the wrist.

2 Repeat movement 1, stopping at the elbow. Lift the receiver's hand and rest it on their opposite shoulder. While you support the elbow, effleurage with your right hand from elbow to shoulder. Finish the movement by stopping at the elbow and letting the receiver's hand relax back down by their left side.

3 Complete the arm massage by repeating movement 1.

4 Cover the left arm with a towel to keep it warm, and repeat the above sequence on the right arm.

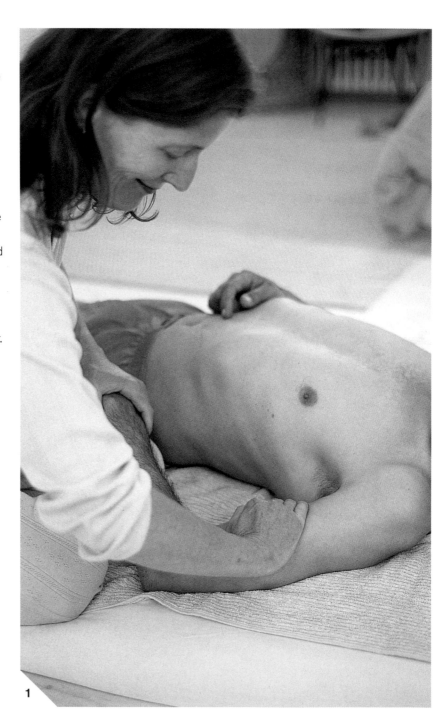

1

Chest and neck

Positioning yourself at the receiver's head, massage oil over the chest, behind the shoulders, drawing up to the back of the neck into the hairline. Pin back the receiver's hair if necessary. Repeat the sequence four times.

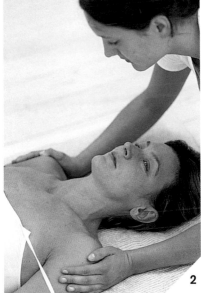

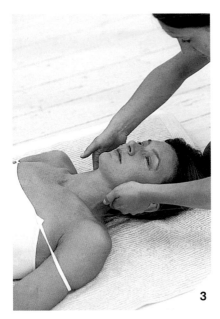

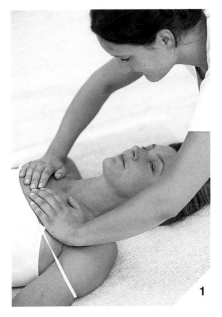

2 Continue the movement by stroking your hands behind the shoulders towards the back of the neck.

3 With slight pressure, draw your hands into the back of the neck and gently pull into the hairline.

4 Relax the fingers back onto the upper chest.

1 Place your hands palm down with your fingers pointing towards the receiver's feet. Gently effleurage your hands away from each other towards the shoulders.

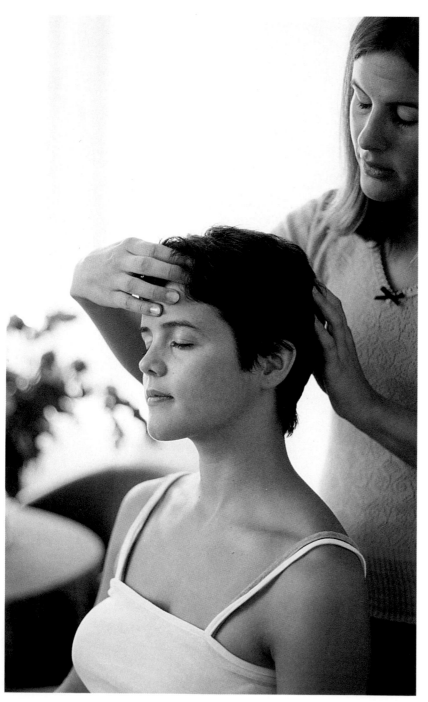

Face

It is important to use confident, firm strokes when massaging the face. This facial massage will help to relieve tension and headaches. The massage will also increase the circulation, which will improve the complexion and give a healthy glow. Apply oil to your hands and stand at the head of the receiver. Repeat each of the following movements four times.

1 Starting with the upper chest, using alternate hands, gently sweep from the shoulder to the jawbone, starting at the left side and finishing at the right side of the jaw.

2 Finish this movement when your right hand meets the jaw at the right side of the face. Your left hand is now ready to cup the jaw and sweep to the opposite side of the face. Repeat with your right hand to cup the jaw and sweep to the left side of the face. Repeat, sweeping left to right several times.

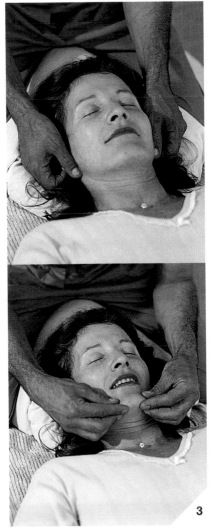

3 To begin the next movement, finish with both fingertips at each end of the jaw with fingers resting lightly under the earlobe. Draw the fingers down to the chin, following the jawline. Bring the fingers up the side of the nose, then across the cheekbone, to form a triangle on the cheeks.

4 Continue by drawing the fingers from the chin up towards the nose. Stroke up the nose and continue to the forehead.

5 Stroke the forehead with alternate palms of the hands, moving from the right to the left side of the forehead.

6 Finish the movement by circling round the eyes using the ring finger.

7 To finish the face massage, gently place the heel of your hands over the eyes with your fingers extending downwards. Hold for 10 seconds.

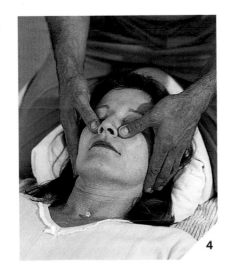

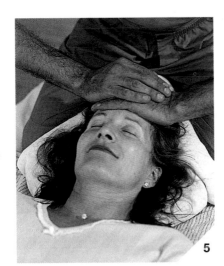

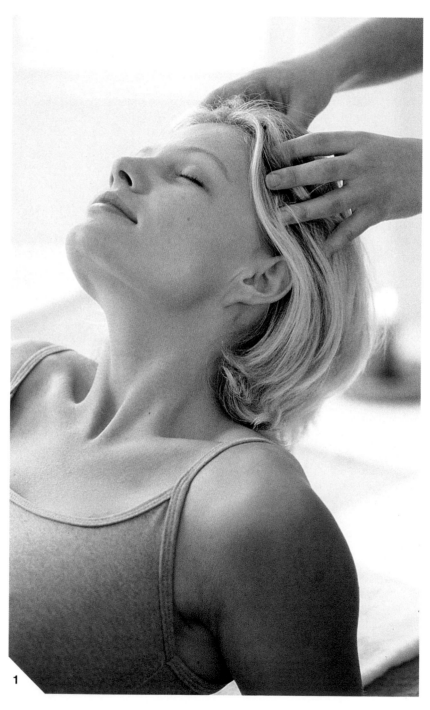

1

Scalp

There is no need to apply more oil, as there will be enough residue on your hands to complete the scalp massage. Repeat each of the following movements four times.

1 Place your hands behind the neck and, with light firm pressure, using thumbs and fingers, make circular friction movements through the hair and all over the scalp. You may find that it helps to move the receiver's head from side to side in order to massage the entire scalp.

2 Gently stroke through the hair, allowing your fingertips to brush the scalp.

3 Finish the movement by lightly moving off at the very tips of the hair, and gently placing your fingertips on the forehead of the receiver. Hold your hands in this position for several seconds while you wish the receiver good thoughts.

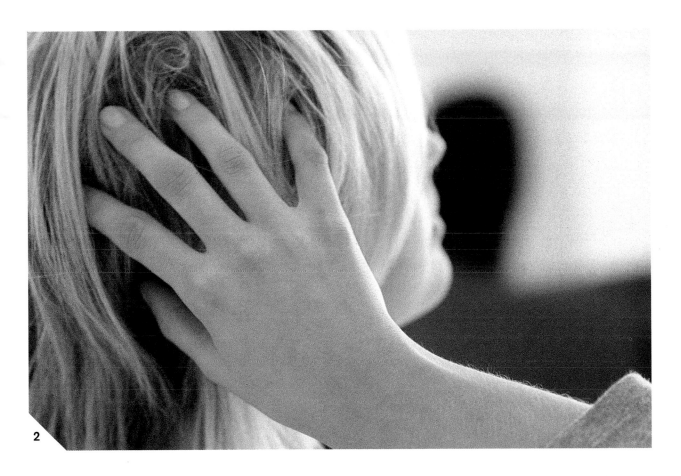

2

Finishing the massage

Quietly cover the receiver with the towels. Place your right hand over the receiver's abdomen and your left hand on the crown of their head. Encourage them to take two or three deep breaths, and to exhale with a sigh. Hold your hands in this position for a few seconds, allowing the receiver to breathe normally. When you are ready, quietly move away, allowing the receiver to rest for a while and to 'come round' in their own time. When the receiver is ready to get up, give them a warm drink.

Sensual massage

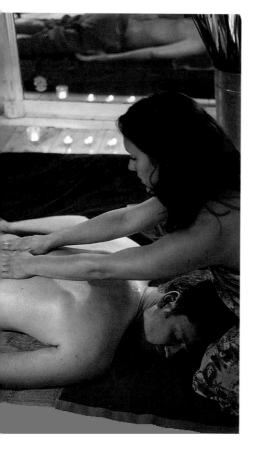

A clinical aromatherapy massage performed by a qualified therapist is for the purpose of creating deep relaxation and self-healing. Sensual aromatherapy, on the other hand, is for anyone who wishes to work with their partner to enhance an erotic massage which will tease and awaken desire. The movements for this massage are very slow and rhythmic, and are based on effleurage, feathering and kneading (see page 30). Attention is drawn to

the erogenous zones of the body: the soles of the feet and in between the toes and fingers, the backs of the knees and the insides of the thighs, the buttocks, the lower back, the breasts, the palms, the insides of the elbows, the armpits, the back of the neck, the ears and finally the lips.

Generally, what feels good for you will also feel good for your lover. However, the ancient erotic texts proclaim that women are more responsive to gentle and lingering movements while men prefer firmer stimulation. You will need to discover together what you and your lover find erotic. Never be afraid to ask; you know what you enjoy and your partner should be only too happy to pleasure you.

To provide a sensual massage, follow the massage sequence described on pages 34–47, but with the following variations.

Back

Standing at your lover's head, place your hands on either side of the uppermost part of the spine, with fingers pointing towards the buttocks. With firm pressure, using effleurage, move your hands down the length of the back and over the buttocks. Effleurage out over the buttocks towards the hips, and slide up each side of the body to the armpits. Slowly continue the

effleurage down over the arms to the hands and entwine your hands and fingers with your partner's. Hold this for a few seconds, allowing your breath to caress your lover's back and shoulders. Feel the warmth and the love within yourself. Slowly draw your fingers away and caress the inside of your partner's arms back towards the shoulder to begin the movement again.

Essential oils beneficial for sensual massage:

Clary sage is exhilarating and euphoric to the mind, creating a heady and warm feeling.
Patchouli helps to increase sexual desire.
Vetiver is a grounding oil that helps to relieve tension and allows relaxation.
Ylang ylang has aphrodisiac qualities that are beneficial in increasing sexual desire.

Try the following sensual massage blend:
* 15ml (½fl oz) sunflower carrier oil
* 2 drops clary sage
* 1 drop patchouli
* 1 drop vetiver
* 2 drops ylang ylang

Stomach and chest

Gently rest your fingers, which are pointing downwards, on your partner's shoulders. With light pressure, slide your hands very slowly over the breast or chest, down towards the abdomen and the pubic bone. Fan your hands, and effleurage out to either side of the hips, slightly cupping the side of the body with your hands, then draw your hands back slowly up either side of the body towards the armpit. On reaching the armpit, bring your right hand over

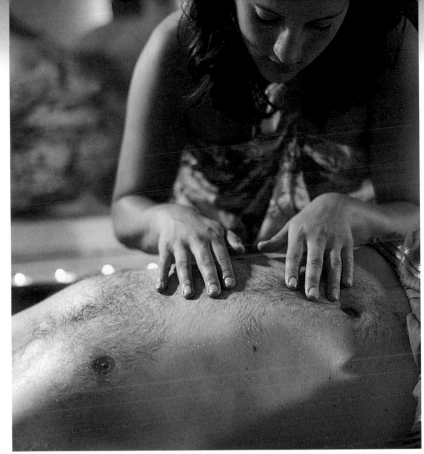

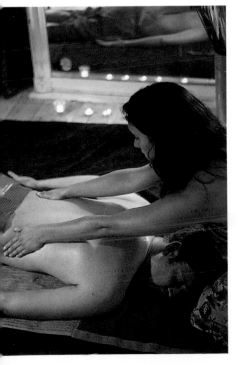

to join your left hand. Place the fingers of your left hand underneath your partner's back.

Start the movement by lifting the muscle from the back and pulling upwards towards the breast and chest area, then repeat the movement by placing your right hand underneath your partner's back and slide forward, picking up the skin. The hands work alternately by picking up the muscle from the back and releasing when reaching the chest area. Repeat on the other side.

Finish by effleurage circling around the outer breast area, and be ready to start the whole movement again from the top of the chest. Repeat the movement as many times as you wish.

Ears

When massaging the scalp, add ear caressing by lightly circling each ear with your fingertips. Gently knead and pull the earlobe between finger and thumb. Finish by feather touching through the hair.

To finish

When finishing any massage movement, always feather stroke the body or part of body that you are working on. Then slowly and gently lift the fingertips away. Light feather stroking will send your partner into orbit and leave them floating in a world of sensuous feelings.

Massage for babies and children

In parts of eastern Asia, and in many tropical countries, baby massage is regarded as one of the essential skills of parenthood. Oiling, stroking and stretching the body is believed to help babies grow stronger by encouraging deep sleep, better feeding, relief of colic and bonding with the parent.

Learning to massage babies and older children can be an important building-block that leads to genuine empathy and love between parent and child. Once a child is used to a massage routine, and it becomes part of a daily or weekly routine, then he or she will associate the massage with a parent's total attention and recognize it as a valuable gift of love. Massage from an early age can nurture feelings of confidence and positive self-image. It also helps if siblings are taught to give massage as well as to receive it, because this encourages harmony and tolerance in the household and mutual respect.

How the child benefits

In a study in a hospital in England, it was shown that babies in incubators developed their lung capacity much more quickly if they were touched or stroked by their parents than if they were just handled by a nurse or left alone in their incubators. Gentle massage on the abdomen can help alleviate problems with the digestive

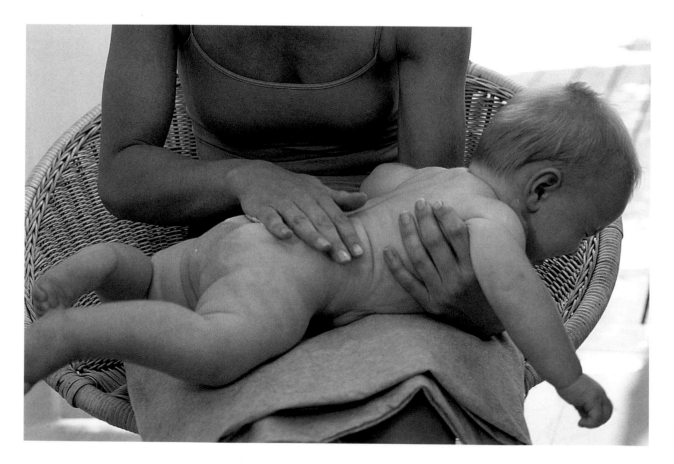

system, such as constipation, diarrhoea or nausea. Massage also helps to promote a healthy mind-body relationship in a developing child.

Baby massage

Much can be achieved by giving up five minutes of your time to massage your baby. If the baby loves it, give them more time; 10–15 minutes is usually long enough for most babies. Make sure the room is warm and, if massaging on the floor, free from draughts. You can begin by stroking your baby lightly with sunflower oil. Try to massage your baby every day, perhaps just before bathtime and at least half an hour after a feed. As your baby grows a little older, he or she will take an active part in the massage by wriggling, kicking and gurgling in response to your touch. So be relaxed and enjoy the game between you.

It may be best to sit on the floor with your legs outstretched, or sit back on your heels. Sit in whatever position is comfortable for you. Leave plenty of space and padding for the baby to move around easily. As a baby's body is so small, you will tend to use mostly stroking and stretching movements, as described here. The massage does not need to be done 'by the book', however – just do whatever your baby enjoys.

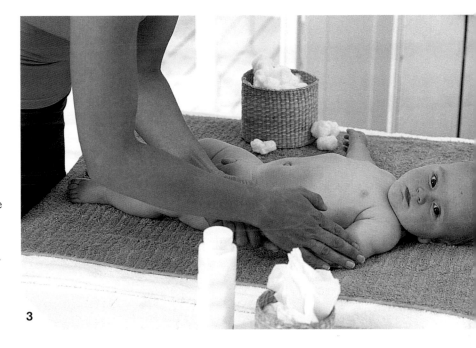

3

Simple baby-massage techniques

1 Begin on the front of the body. Apply a little massage oil with long strokes all over the baby's body. Stroke the baby from shoulders to feet, but avoid the face to prevent the possibility of the oil seeping into the eyes.

2 Massage the baby's tummy with your fingertips, stroking clockwise around the navel.

3 Hold the baby's hand in one of your hands, gently stretching the limb. Stroke the entire arm from shoulder to wrist, then squeeze all the way down the arm. Repeat several times. Now massage the other arm.

4 Hold the baby's foot and gently stretch the limb. Stroke the leg from thigh to ankle, then squeeze the leg all the way down. Repeat several times. Massage the other leg.

5 Turn the baby over and oil the back of the body.

6 Begin by stroking the legs, over the buttocks and up the back. Slide your hands across the shoulders and down the arms, and then glide them down the sides of the baby's body to the feet. Repeat this movement several times.

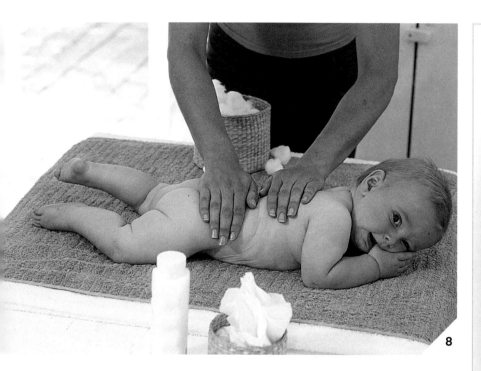

8

Essential oils beneficial for babies and children:

Roman camomile is a peaceful oil with soothing properties, promoting relaxation. Its analgesic action eases pain, whether it is caused by colic or toothache. It is also helpful with eczema or dry and itchy skin, and allergic conditions generally. **Lavender** is an excellent sedative oil with pain-relieving qualities. Its anti-viral properties make it useful for the respiratory system; it is also an invaluable oil for all skin conditions.

Sunflower oil is a good carrier oil to use on babies and children as it has a softening and moisturizing effect on the skin.

For babies under 3 years old, add 1 drop of Roman camomile or lavender to 50ml (2fl oz) of sunflower oil. If both essential oils are required, blend the Roman camomile and lavender together and take 1 drop from the mix.

7 Babies love having their bottoms patted, so with four fingers of one hand gently pat the buttocks. Stroke over and around each buttock, then very gently press the buttocks together.

8 Finish the back by sliding your hands very gently and smoothly down the baby's back, one hand following the other. As one hand reaches the legs, lift it off, return the hand to the top of the back and repeat the movement. Gradually stroke more and more slowly and lightly. This smooth, continuous stroke will have a calming effect on your baby.

9 After the massage, wrap your baby in a warm towel. He or she will probably fall asleep, or just lie in your arms for a while.

Aromatherapy for older children

Children of all ages benefit from the use of essential oils. The massage movements for children are the same as for adults, but when you make a blend for the massage mix remember to follow the guidelines of 2 drops of essential oil in 20ml (¾fl oz) of carrier base oil, and use only 2 drops of the essential oil in the bath.

Caution: Essential oils are very powerful and care should always be taken when using them on children.

Cuts and bruises
Young children frequently fall over and receive minor cuts and bruises to their skin. The essential oils fight infection and can be used to promote the healing of wounds. Essential oils that are beneficial for these types of cuts and bruises are lavender, lemon, niaouli and tea tree. Use 2 drops of any one of these essential oils in your child's bath.

Insomnia
Parents need their children to sleep at night so that they themselves can get some rest and be energized for the next day. Insomnia in children can have many causes, ranging from over-excitedness, fearfulness or, in the case of young children, missing the comfort of their parents'

company. A warm bath at night using essential oils will help the winding-down process.

✳ For over-excited children who go to bed and cannot relax, blend 1 drop each of lavender and ylang ylang into 20ml (¾fl oz) of sunflower base oil and massage their back. Using gentle effleurage strokes, with the flat of your hand start at the bottom of the back and slide up either side of the spine, up over the shoulders and around the shoulder blades. Keep repeating this movement, and, as you see the child relax, allow your pressure to become lighter and lighter, then lift your hand off, leaving at the fingertips. This movement will totally relax your child, and will be something comforting and pleasant for them to look forward to when they go to bed. It will only take a few minutes.

✳ A blend for the fearful or worrying child is 1 drop each of frankincense and lavender into 20ml (¾fl oz) of sunflower oil, using the same massage movement as above.

✳ Children who cannot sleep because they miss the comfort of their parents will benefit if their parents, during the day, wear a perfume blend of lavender and

sweet orange. At night, when the child is ready for bed, put some of the perfume mix used by the parents on a soft cuddly toy and place it beside your child. The smell will comfort the child and give them a sense of security.

Common ailments

This section is divided into various types of ailment: problems with the respiratory system, the circulatory system, the digestive system, the immune system, the female reproductive system, muscles and bones and the skin. For each ailment, recommendations are made for essential oils, synergistic blends, carrier bases and methods of use.

When combining an essential oil with a carrier base, always use 2 drops of essential oil only. For synergistic blends, follow the individual recommendations.

If more than one carrier oil is suggested, these should be blended together before adding the essential oil.

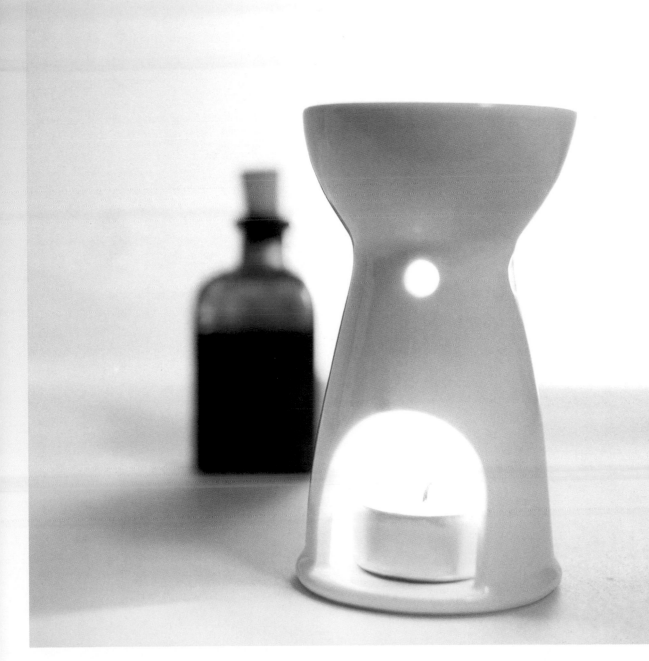

Respiratory system

Life depends on the ability to breathe in oxygen and to eliminate carbon dioxide. Breathing is the movement of air in and out of the lungs. When sitting quietly, a person breathes in and out about 12–15 times a minute; during excessive exercise, that rate can be trebled. Respiration is the exchange of oxygen and carbon dioxide between the atmosphere and the cells of the body. It involves a chemical process inside the cells whereby food substances are oxidized to produce energy and the waste product carbon dioxide is eliminated from the system.

Coughing

We cough for two reasons:

✳ Insufficient mucus. This is often seen in allergic and asthmatic conditions and in dry, irritating coughs. The mucus is too sticky to flow adequately. If the problem is prolonged, congestion may occur and chronic bronchitis can result.

✳ Too much mucus. This is otherwise known as catarrhal condition. Excessive mucus overloads the ciliary mechanism, leading to congestion. Bronchitis and other lung infections can occur as a result.

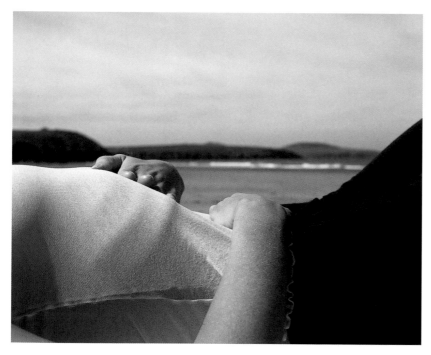

Respiratory ailments

Respiratory ailments affect the mucous membranes. These include the linings of the nasal passage, the larynx, the pharynx, the trachea and the lungs, which consist of the bronchial tubes, bronchioles and the alveoli sacs. When in good health, we are not aware of respiratory mucus, which is swept downwards into the sterilizing stomach by the action of the beating cilia. Cilia are microscopic hairs that grow from the cells lining the air passages, and which wave backwards and forwards. When we become run down, our immunity level drops and we are unable to resist airborne bacteria and viruses. The mucus becomes more viscous and is unable to rid itself of these bodies of toxins, which have become congested and can lead to chronic catarrh. We then begin to cough in an attempt by the body's natural response to rid ourselves of this excess.

Asthma

Symptoms and causes

Asthma can trigger off difficulty in breathing, tightness in the chest and wheezing and coughing caused by excessive mucus. Possible causes are allergies to, for example, pollen, animal fur, fungi and dairy products. Emotional stress can also play a part.

Recommended essential oils

Clary sage has a euphoric and emotionally uplifting quality. It strengthens the defence system and aids recovery after illness.

Cypress relaxes spasms in the bronchial tubes, which helps coughs associated with asthma.

Frankincense has a pronounced effect on the mucous membranes, and is particularly helpful in clearing the lungs. It calms the emotions and eases shortness of breath.

Other useful essential oils

Clary sage, cypress, eucalyptus (*Eucalyptus globulus, E. smithii*), frankincense, galbanum, lavender, Spanish marjoram, true melissa, myrrh, bitter orange, peppermint, sandalwood, tea tree and sweet thyme.

Synergistic blend
❋ 2 drops clary sage
❋ 2 drops cypress
❋ 2 drops frankincense

Massage carrier base
❋ 15ml (½fl oz) sunflower oil

Methods of use
❋ Bathing
❋ Dry inhalation (drops on a handkerchief)
❋ Regular massages to chest, neck and shoulders (see page 43)

Caution: Do not inhale with hot steam. It may take the breath away.

Herbal tradition
Clary sage was called 'clear eye' by medieval herbalists, who used it to alleviate eye complaints.

Cypress was highly valued by ancient civilizations as a medicine, and is still used by the Tibetans as purification incense.

Frankincense, a sweet-smelling resin from Arabia, is mentioned in the Bible. It was one of the gifts presented by the three wise men to the newborn Jesus.

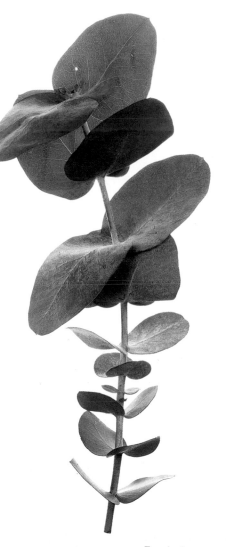

Eucalyptus
(*Eucalyptus globulus*)

Bronchitis

Symptoms and causes

Bronchitis is an infection of the bronchial tubes that leads to the lungs. This can bring on symptoms of a chesty cough, chest pain, aching muscles and irritation between the shoulder blades, with a high temperature. Depression may also be a symptom. Possible causes are incorrect breathing, air pollution, allergy, stress and excessive consumption of dairy products and/or junk food. Often there is a complication of a bacterial infection facilitated by viral inflammation.

Sweet thyme

Recommended essential oils

Cajuput is an excellent antiseptic for the respiratory tract. It is particularly beneficial at the start of an infection, and for the irritation often found with acute bronchitis. It increases perspiration which helps to minimize feverish temperatures and release flu toxins from the body.

Sandalwood is a useful oil for chest infections, sore throats and dry coughs which accompany bronchitis and lung infections. It aids sleep when catarrhal conditions are present and helps to stimulate the immune system.

Sweet thyme (*Thymus vulgaris* ct. *geraniol* ct. *linalol*) stimulates the action of white corpuscles, helping the body fight infection, and deters the spread of germs.

Synergistic blend

✳ 2 drops cajuput
✳ 1 drop sandalwood
✳ 3 drops sweet thyme

Massage carrier base

✳ 15ml (½fl oz) sunflower oil

Methods of use

✳ Steam inhalation
✳ Vaporizing
✳ Bathing
✳ Chest and back rub
✳ Massage back and shoulder
   blades by placing your hands

either side of the spine at the base of the back and effleurage up towards the shoulders. Proceed in a figure of eight around the shoulder blades. Relax your hands back down to the starting point to begin again. This will help relax the tension in the back and break down the congestion.

Herbal tradition

Cajuput grows wild in Malaysia, where it is called *caju-puti*, meaning 'white wood', due to the colour of the timber. It is used locally for colds, throat infections, headaches and muscle fatigue.

Sandalwood is the oldest known perfume material and has been in continuous use for over 4,000 years, traditionally used as incense or for embalming bodies.

Other useful essential oils

Bay, cajuput, cedarwood (Atlas and Virginian), cypress, frankincense, ginger, immortelle, lavender, myrrh, niaouli, sandalwood and sweet thyme.

Sinusitis

Symptoms and causes

This is an infection of the hollow sinus cavities, resulting in congestion, pain around the eyes, headaches and halitosis. Possible causes are stress, food allergy and air pollution. It can be triggered by a cold or flu.

Recommended essential oils

Immortelle is a general aid to the respiratory system, soothing feverish colds, coughs, bronchitis and sinusitis. It boosts the immune system and helps keep allergies and infections at bay. It also helps to remove mucus from the lungs and induces relaxation and sleep.

Lemon relieves headaches and migraine caused by sinusitis, as well as neuralgic pain. It stimulates the white corpuscles, thereby invigorating the immune system and aiding the body in fighting infections.

Myrtle seems to have a pronounced clearing effect on sinusitis. Although it resembles eucalyptus in action, it does not possess the same stimulating properties. The sedative properties of myrtle make it very beneficial at night.

Synergistic blend

* 1 drop immortelle
* 2 drops lemon
* 3 drops myrtle

Herbal tradition

Lemon was used in ancient times to perfume clothes and repel insects. It was later used to help sailors combat scurvy while at sea for long periods.

Myrtle was used by the Greek physician Dioscorides, who lived in Anazarbus (which is now known as south central Turkey) and who was a surgeon with the Roman army during the reign of emperor Nero. He prescribed it for clearing the lungs, and gave it in a form of extract made by macerating the leaves in wine.

Facial massage carrier base

* 15ml (½fl oz) sunflower oil

Methods of use

* Bathing
* Steam inhalation
* Dry inhalation (2 drops of the above blend on a tissue)
* Vaporizing
* Facial massage. Using the above blend, place the ring fingers under the inside corners of the eyebrows. Slide the fingers to the outer corner of the eye, lifting the brow at the same time. When you have reached the outer corner of the

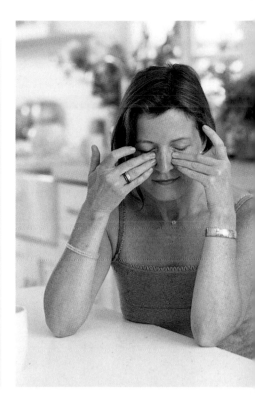

eye, continue the movement with the third finger, sliding it along the cheekbone to a point under the centre of the eye. Slide the fingers back to the starting point and repeat the motion.

Other useful essential oils

Cajuput, eucalyptus (*Eucalyptus globulus, E. smithii*), lavender, niaouli, peppermint, pine, tea tree and sweet thyme.

Circulatory system

The circulatory system is made up of the heart, arteries, arterioles, capillaries, veins and blood. The basic function of the circulatory system is to ensure that blood reaches all parts of the body. Every cell must receive nourishment, which is provided by the blood. The circulatory system also ensures that the waste products of the cells – carbon dioxide, urea and lactic acid – are carried to the kidneys, intestines, lungs and skin, where they are excreted.

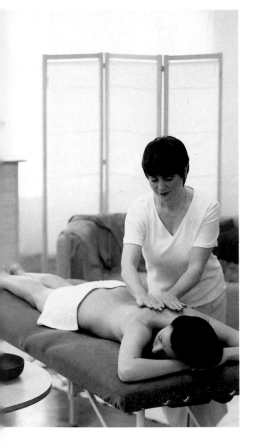

Evidence shows that lifestyle is a contributing factor to the disease process. Two-thirds of all deaths in Western society are attributable to problems with the circulatory system. Risk factors, such as cigarette smoking, excess intake of salt, saturated fats and refined processed foods, excessive alcohol and lack of exercise, can all aid the onslaught of the disease.

The vitality and tone of the circulatory system are fundamental to life and to the integration of all the parts of the body. Any breakdown in this system will have a profound effect on the tissues and organs involved. The blood may be healthy, but if the supply of blood to the organs is not adequate there will be problems. Likewise, if waste materials produced in the metabolic process are not removed, damage to tissues will result.

Preventative measures

Prevention of circulatory problems is much better than having to resort to curing a disease that has developed. This can be achieved by giving up smoking, taking adequate exercise, eating sensibly, maintaining an average weight for your build and reducing the stress in your life. Aromatherapy places great emphasis upon preventative care. Massaging with aromatic oils reigns supreme within the complementary therapies as being most beneficial for circulation and stress-related conditions.

Caution: Never use massage in cases of thrombosis or phlebitis, as it could dislodge or move the blood clots which are present.

High blood pressure

Symptoms and causes

Blood pressure rises as a result of an increase in resistance to the flow of blood in both large and small blood vessels. About 90 per cent of people with hypertension have no obvious underlying cause for their elevated blood pressure; this is called essential hypertension. Possible causes for essential hypertension can be prolonged stress, smoking, alcohol, a sedentary lifestyle and obesity. For the other 10 per cent, a definite cause is found; this is called secondary hypertension.

Specific causes can be disorders of the adrenal glands or the kidneys, a complication of pregnancy or a type of congenital heart defect. Severe hypertension may sometimes cause shortness of breath, giddiness and visual disturbances.

Caution: The following oils are contraindicated for high blood pressure: hyssop, rosemary, common sage and red thyme. Always seek professional help for high blood pressure. Using aromatherapy and self-help remedies may be beneficial for mild cases, but do not replace long-term blood pressure medication with aromatherapy remedies without first consulting your doctor.

Recommended essential oils

Bergamot has a sedative yet uplifting character which is excellent for anxiety, depression and treating nervous tension.

Neroli is rather hypnotic and euphoric, and will soothe emotional states and relive chronic anxiety, depression and stress.

Ylang ylang is an excellent oil for excitable conditions, regulating the adrenaline flow and relaxing the nervous system. It eases feelings of panic, anxiety and fear.

Synergistic blend
✳ 2 drops bergamot
✳ 1 drop neroli
✳ 3 drops ylang ylang

Massage carrier base
✳ 15ml (½fl oz) sunflower oil

Methods of use
✳ Bathing
✳ Full body massage
✳ Vaporizing
✳ Personal perfume

Other useful essential oils
Roman camomile, frankincense, lavender, sweet marjoram, neroli and rose otto.

Herbal tradition
Bergamot is an ingredient in Earl Grey tea and provides its distinctive flavour.

Neroli, also known as orange blossom, is named after the 17th-century princess from Nerola who introduced the oil to Italian society. It has been used variously by prostitutes in Madrid and in bridal bouquets to denote purity in folk culture.

Ylang ylang has aphrodisiac qualities, and in Indonesia its petals are strewn on the marriage bed of newlyweds.

Cellulite

Symptoms and causes

Cellulite is an accumulation of water and toxic wastes in the connective tissue surrounding the fat cells. The tissue around the fat cells tends to harden, imprisoning the water and causing unsightly bulges. Possible causes can be a hormonal imbalance, poor circulation, unbalanced diet, abuse of tea, coffee, cigarettes or alcohol, and stress.

Recommended essential oils

Grapefruit is a lymphatic stimulant, and with its excellent diuretic properties helps eliminate water and toxic waste from the bodily systems.

Juniper berry is well known for its detoxifying properties. It clears the body of toxins, particularly when too much alcohol and rich food has been consumed.

Red thyme *(Thymus vulgaris* ct. *thymol)* is good for the circulation, and its stimulating and diuretic action facilitates the removal of uric acid.

Synergistic blend
✳ 2 drops grapefruit
✳ 2 drops juniper berry
✳ 2 drops red thyme

Massage carrier base
✳ 10ml (⅙fl oz) grapeseed oil
✳ 5ml avocado oil

Methods of use
✳ Regular lymphatic massage (see page 35)
✳ Bathing
✳ Self-massage (see page 31)

Herbal tradition

Juniper, with its pine-fresh scent, has long been valued for its antiseptic properties. The ancient Greeks used it to fight epidemics, and during medieval times crushed juniper berries were added to hot baths to treat respiratory infections.

Common thyme is one of the earliest medicinal plants employed throughout the Mediterranean region. It was used by the ancient Egyptians in the embalming process and by the ancient Greeks to fumigate against infectious illness. The name thyme derives from the Greek word *thymos*, meaning 'to perfume'.

Other useful essential oils

Carrot seed, cypress, fennel, geranium, ginger, lemon, bitter orange and rosemary.

Red thyme (*Thymus vulgaris* ct. *thymol*)

Fluid retention

Symptoms and causes

Fluid retention usually causes swelling of the feet and ankles. Possible causes are pre-menstrual tension, standing or sitting for too long, injury to the body (which can cause the body to retain fluid) and lack of exercise.

Recommended essential oils

Carrot seed is an excellent purifier of the body, mainly due to its detoxifying effect on the liver, and it helps reduce fluid retention.

Geranium has a stimulating effect on the

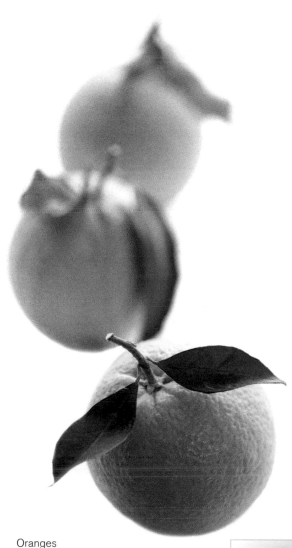

Oranges

Herbal tradition

Carrot seed has been traditionally used for the retention of urine, colic, kidney and digestive disorders. In Chinese traditional medicine, it is used to treat dysentery and to expel worms.

Geranium has a floral, exotic aroma, and is sometimes used as an aphrodisiac.

Oranges are given as Chinese New Year gifts to promote happiness and prosperity.

lymphatic system, which disposes of waste products and water. It is also a tonic to the circulation, as it makes it more fluid.

Sweet orange is a lymphatic stimulant that helps reduce toxic waste and water retention.

Synergistic blend
* 1 drop carrot seed
* 3 drops geranium
* 2 drops sweet orange

Massage carrier base
* 15ml (½fl oz) grapeseed oil

Other useful essential oils
Cypress, fennel, grapefruit, juniper berry, mandarin and rosemary.

Digestive system

We need food to live. Health and vitality depend on the digestive system's ability to provide nutrients for the body. The digestive system begins with the mouth and ends with the rectum. The system is an amazing 11m (36ft) long. The digestive system prepares food for use and distribution through the following five basic activities:

✳ Taking food into the body by eating.
✳ Moving the food along the digestive tract.
✳ Breaking down food by both mechanical and chemical processes.
✳ Absorbing the nutrients into the bloodstream for distribution to the cells.
✳ Eliminating indigestible substances from the body.

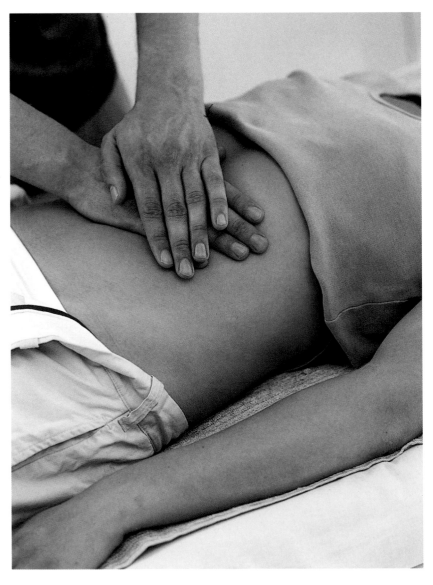

Balancing the emotions

The functions and health of the digestive system are closely related to our emotional state. Sometimes when we feel a strong emotion, such as stress, fear or anger, we experience a 'gut reaction'. Emotional anxiety causes the stomach to produce excess acid. This feeling may just be for a moment, but if it continues, the prolonged anger, fear or stress can lead to disturbances within the digestive system, such as diminished appetite, constipation, heartburn, diarrhoea and nausea.

If the emotional problem becomes chronic, problems such as gastric ulcers or irritable bowel syndrome (IBS) can occur. It is important, therefore, to eat a healthy diet and live a balanced lifestyle to avoid serious digestive problems.

Irritable bowel syndrome (IBS)

Symptoms and causes

Irritable bowel syndrome is known for a range of symptoms associated with poor digestive function. Sufferers experience abdominal pain, bloating, constipation or diarrhoea, flatulence and nausea. Stools may contain mucus and blood, and can resemble small, hard rabbit droppings. Possible causes of IBS include stress and food intolerance.

Recommended essential oils

Sweet marjoram is known for its soothing effect on the digestive system, relieving cramps, indigestion, constipation and flatulence, and aiding the clearing of toxins.

Black pepper has a fortifying effect on the stomach, increases the flow of saliva, expels wind and subdues nausea. It is useful in bowel problems because it gives general tone to the colon muscles.

Peppermint benefits all types of acute conditions associated with the digestive system. It has a beneficial action on the stomach, liver and intestines. Its antispasmodic action relieves the smooth muscles of the stomach and gut, helping stomach pain, colic, diarrhoea, indigestion, halitosis, gallstones and vomiting.

Synergistic blend
✳ 2 drops sweet marjoram
✳ 2 drops black pepper
✳ 2 drops peppermint

Massage carrier base
✳ 15ml (½fl oz) grapeseed oil

Methods of use
✳ Gently massage the abdomen in a clockwise direction
✳ Compress
✳ Bathing
✳ Full body massage

Herbal tradition
Black peppercorns were traditionally used in Greece for fever and to fortify the stomach. In India, holy men used to swallow whole grains of pepper to give them the stamina for walking long distances.

Sweet marjoram was much prized by the ancient Egyptians, who placed it on the graves of the dead to aid them in the afterlife.

Peppermint settles the stomach and is also believed to stimulate the brain.

Handy hint
Take peppermint oil capsules (these are available from health-food shops).

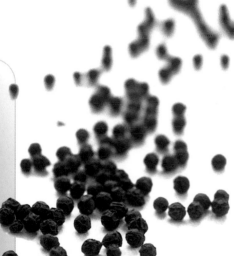

Black pepper

Other useful essential oils
Roman camomile, fennel, lavender, mandarin and neroli.

Travel sickness

Symptoms and causes

When travelling, you may experience a sudden need to vomit, which makes you feel hot and sticky, and is followed by stomach cramps. Travel sickness is to a large extent caused by conflicting messages reaching the brain from the eyes and from the balancing mechanism of the ears and the stomach.

Recommended essential oils

Cardamom is beneficial for a nervous stomach. Its calmative properties act as a laxative and deal with colic, wind and that uncomfortable feeling in the upper digestive tract. It also eases feelings of nausea.

Fennel is an excellent tonic for the digestive system, working on ailments such as indigestion caused by stress, nausea, vomiting and colic.

Ginger is a calmative oil that is especially effective against the feeling of nausea, hangovers and travel sickness.

Synergistic blend

❋ 2 drops cardamom
❋ 2 drops fennel
❋ 2 drops ginger

Method of use

❋ Dry inhalation (2 drops on a handkerchief or tissue)

Other useful essential oils

Coriander, lavender and peppermint.

Herbal tradition

In ancient Greece, it was believed that fennel provided strength and courage, and it was consumed by athletes to improve their performance. In medieval times, fennel was thought to ward off witches. Ginger has been used for thousands of years, especially in the East. Fresh ginger is used in China for many complaints including rheumatism, diarrhoea, malaria and colds. In the West, it is best known as a digestive aid.

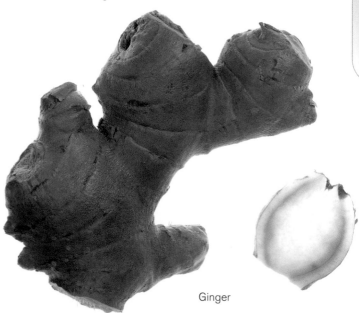

Ginger

Indigestion

Symptoms and causes

Indigestion is a common term covering a variety of symptoms brought on by eating too much or too quickly, or eating very rich, spicy or fatty foods. Nervous indigestion is a common effect of stress.

Caution: *Anyone with severe or persistent pain, weight loss or vomiting, or who develops resistant diarrhoea or constipation, should consult a doctor immediately.*

Recommended essential oils

Cinnamon leaf calms spasms of the digestive tract, indigestion, diarrhoea, colitis, vomiting and nausea.

Coriander has a soothing, warming effect on the stomach, relieving wind and stomach cramps. It has been known to help with eating disorders.

Handy hint

When the symptoms begin, blend the synergistic oils with the carrier oil and, starting from the right side of the stomach, massage the stomach in a circular movement. This will help release trapped wind and relieve cramped muscles.

Herbal tradition

Coriander is a herb with a long history of use; the seeds were found in the ancient Egyptian tomb of Rameses II.

❊

Cinnamon was traded by Arabs in the middle ages. They maintained their monopoly of the spice trade by claiming that cinnamon was harvested from the nests of ferocious birds and had to be gathered under their attack.

❊

Bitter orange The flowers from the bitter orange tree were used in bridal bouquets and wreaths, to calm any nervous apprehension before the couple retired to the marriage bed.

Other useful essential oils

Angelica, cardamom, camomile (German and Roman), fennel, ginger, mandarin, sweet marjoram, neroli, black pepper, and peppermint.

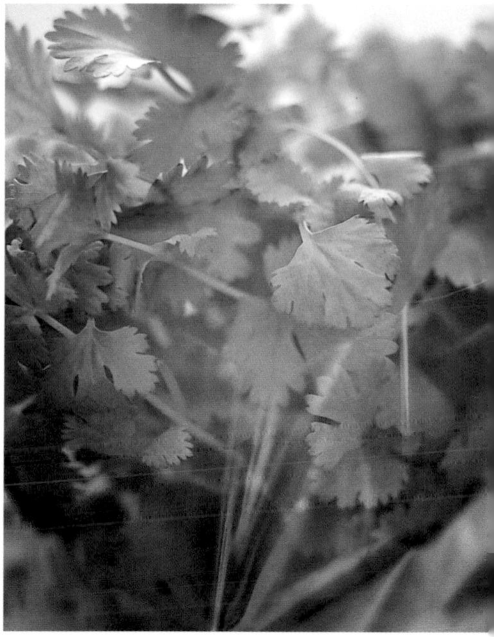

Coriander

Bitter orange seems to have a calming action on the stomach, especially in nervous states. It can help by stimulating bile and could help with the digestion of fats.

Synergistic blend

- 1 drop cinnamon leaf
- 2 drops coriander
- 2 drops bitter orange

Massage carrier base

- 15ml (½fl oz) grapeseed oil

Methods of use

- Full body massage
- Warm compress

Immune system

The immune system consists of a group of cells, molecules and organs which act together to defend the body against foreign invaders that may cause disease, such as bacteria, viruses and fungi. The health of the body is dependent on the immune system's ability to recognize and then repel or destroy these invaders. Immune proficiency is provided and maintained by two cellular systems, which involve lymphocytes. Lymphocytes are cells produced by the body's primary (bone marrow and thymus) and secondary (lymph nodes and spleen) lymphatic organs.

Stress

There is much evidence to show that immunity and resistances to disease are linked to attitudes, behaviour and emotional states. Research has shown that serious depression can decrease a person's immunity and open them up to infection. Similarly, stress through overworking can also have an adverse effect on the immune system.

In the normal course of events, most people push themselves to the limit and do not give their bodies time to recuperate naturally each day or each week. When they eventually allow themselves some time for a rest or a holiday, the body suddenly relaxes. Because the immune system is not functioning at its best at such a time, the body cannot effectively fight off germs, and illness often results. Most people do not realize the effect their interactions can have on their nervous and immune systems and fail to take the necessary steps to guard against illness.

Auto-immunity

The term 'auto-immunity' literally means immunity against self, and it is a condition caused by a failure of self-tolerance in the body. Failures of the immune system's defences to fight infection can lead to certain deficiencies such as herpes simplex infection or chicken pox, fungal infections, candidiasis (thrush), allergies or hypersensitivity, infectious diseases such as measles, rubella, glandular fever and human immunodeficiency virus (HIV) which can lead on to acquired immune deficiency syndrome (AIDS).

Susceptibility to auto-immune disease has a genetic basis in humans and animals. Numerous viruses, bacteria, chemicals, toxins and drugs have been implicated as the triggering environmental agents in susceptible individuals. The four main causative factors of auto-immune disease are thought to be: genetic predisposition, hormonal influences, infections and stress.

Which oils to use

A weakened immune system will benefit from these types of oils:

✳ Antibiotic and bactericidal, for fighting bacterial infection: basil, elemi, eucalyptus, lemon, lemon grass, myrrh, neroli, niaouli, palmarosa, rose and tea tree.

✳ Anti-viral, for fighting viral infections such as colds and flu: elemi, eucalyptus, immortelle, lavender, spike lavender, palmarosa and tea tree.

✳ Cytophylactic, for increasing the activity of white blood cells: carrot seed, frankincense, geranium, neroli, rose and tagetes.

✳ Detoxifying, for helping cleanse the blood of impurities: fennel, frankincense, juniper berry lavender and black pepper.

✳ Fungicidal, for fighting fungal infections: cedarwood (Atlas and Virginian), immortelle, lavender, lemon grass, myrrh, patchouli, tagetes and tea tree.

✳ Vulnerary, for healing of wounds: benzoin, bergamot, camomile (German and Roman), elemi, eucalyptus, frankincense, geranium, lavender, myrrh, niaouli and rosemary.

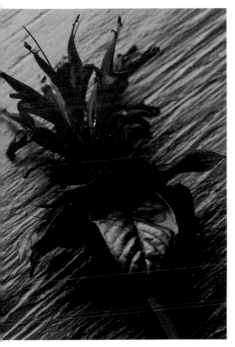

Bergamot

Candida albicans

Symptoms and causes

Candida albicans is a yeast-like fungus that inhabits the stomach, mouth and throat. Normally, it lives in healthy balance in the bowel, but when the body system becomes overworked or stressed, or is recovering from another illness, this fungus takes the opportunity to multiply. This weakens the immune system, which in turn can cause the infection known as candidiasis. The most common symptom is thrush, but candida can lead to nausea, headaches, depression, abnormal fatigue and other fungal outbreaks.

Recommended essential oils

Bergamot is a valuable antiseptic for the urinary tract and is effective at fighting infection and inflammation, most notably cystitis. It is uplifting for the mind and aids the relief of depression.

Eucalyptus *(Eucalyptus citriodora)* has bactericidal and anti-inflammatory properties that make it very powerful against candida and other fungal infections.

Tea tree has fungicidal properties that help clear vaginal thrush, and is of value with genital infections generally.

Synergistic blend
✳ 2 drops bergamot
✳ 2 drops eucalyptus (*E. citriodora*)
✳ 2 drops tea tree

Massage carrier base
✳ Live acidophilus-cultured yogurt (available from health-food stores, this contains an active ingredient that fights candida).

Other useful essential oils
German camomile, lavender, lemon grass, true melissa, myrtle and rosemary.

Method of use
✳ For vaginal thrush, mix the synergistic blend in a 50g (2oz) carton of live yogurt and keep in the refrigerator. Smooth a thin layer of the yogurt mix onto a sanitary towel and wear. Do this once at night and once again the following morning for three days. This mix will help fight the bacteria and will help keep the area cool and take away the itching. (Both partners can use the blend.)

Caution: Do not apply this mix onto a tampon or insert the mixture into the vagina, because this will cause irritation to the mucous membrane.

Herbal tradition
Tea tree derives its name from local usage by the aboriginal people of Australia, who used the leaves as a herbal tea to treat various conditions. In 1770, when Captain Cook landed at Botany Bay, his men discovered the tea tree and also used its sticky leaves to make a spicy drink. It has a strong antiseptic aroma.

Post-viral fatigue syndrome

Symptoms and causes

This condition occurs when you have a low resistance to infection following another illness, and it can cause tiredness, aches and pains. Possible causes are stress, overwork or emotional fatigue.

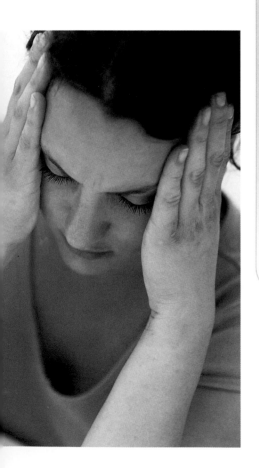

Herbal tradition

Elemi is a tropical tree native to the Philippines, where the gum is used locally for skin care and respiratory complaints. It was also one of the aromatics used by the ancient Egyptians in the embalming process.

Spike lavender is described by the herbalist Nicholas Culpeper (1616–54), in his well-known book *Herbal*. It is recommended for a variety of ailments, including 'pains of the head and brain which proceed form cold, apoplexy, falling sickness, the dropsy or sluggish malady, cramps, convulsions, palsies and often faintings'.

Palmarosa was often used to adulterate rose oil.

Recommended essential oils

Elemi has a strengthening effect on the body through helping it to fight disease. For the mind, it is uplifting and joyous.

Spike lavender builds up the immunity to fight viral attacks and promotes a sense of emotional calm.

Palmarosa is cooling to the body and has a calming but uplifting effect on the emotions.

Synergistic blend
* 1 drop elemi
* 3 drops spike lavender
* 2 drops palmarosa

Massage carrier base
* 15ml (½fl oz) sunflower oil

Methods of use
* Full body massage
* Bathing
* Inhalation
* Vaporizing

Other useful essential oils
Eucalyptus (*Eucalyptus globulus, E. smithii*), immortelle, lavender and tea tree.

Coughs and colds

Symptoms and causes

Colds are caused by a widespread infectious virus causing symptoms of sore throat, stuffy or runny nose, headache, cough and general despondency. One possible reason for catching a cold is a lowered immune system due to overwork and stress.

Recommended essential oils

Benzoin has a good reputation for helping with respiratory disorders. It is a tonic to the lungs and has a beneficial action on coughs, colds and sore throats. This warming oil instils confidence and eases exhausted emotional states.

Peppermint relieves a state of fatigue with its cooling properties. It has a dual action, cooling when hot and warming when cold. This makes it a good cold remedy, halting mucus and fevers, and encouraging perspiration. It clears sinus congestion and relieves headaches with its analgesic properties.

Ravensara is a sedative oil that helps build up the immune system, fight infection and ease coughs.

Synergistic blend
* 1 drop benzoin
* 2 drops peppermint
* 3 drops ravensara

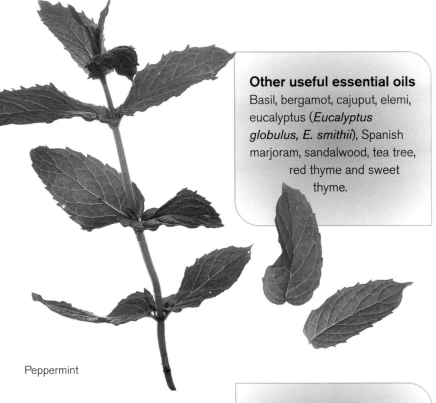

Peppermint

Other useful essential oils
Basil, bergamot, cajuput, elemi, eucalyptus (*Eucalyptus globulus, E. smithii*), Spanish marjoram, sandalwood, tea tree, red thyme and sweet thyme.

Massage carrier base
* 15ml (½fl oz) grapeseed oil

Methods of use
* Facial massage (use the same technique as for sinusitis; see page 59)
* Steam inhalation
* Dry inhalation (2 drops of whole blend on a tissue)

Caution: The essential oils are too strong for direct use on the skin of young children and babies, and can cause seizures if used in inhalation for babies and children.

Herbal tradition
Benzoin has been traditionally used for thousands of years in the East for incense-burning. The fumes from the incense were believed to drive away evil spirits. In the West, it is best known in the form of a compound tincture called 'Friars' balsam', used as a rub for respiratory complaints.

Female reproductive system

Whether we decide to have children or not, the female body is a complex machine designed to make babies. A woman can spend the equivalent of over six years of her life having periods. For some, this means period pain and/or pre-menstrual syndrome. Then, when the fertile years are coming to an end, there is also the menopause to deal with.

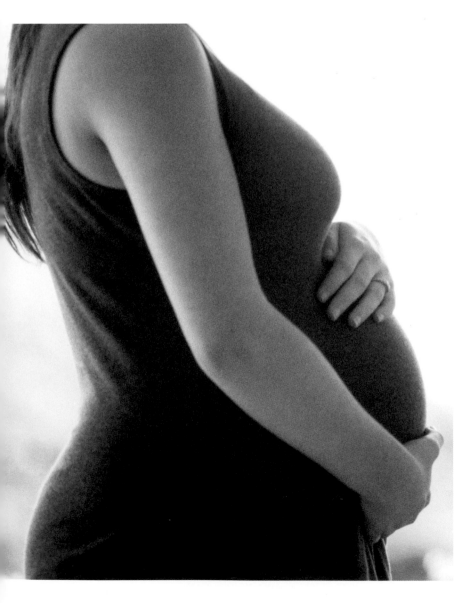

Female hormones and essential oils

The two most important female hormones are oestrogen and progesterone. Oestrogen controls the development and maintenance of the female sexual organs, and gives the women her female shape and physiology. Progesterone prepares the uterine lining for pregnancy each month.

There is evidence that essential oils have hormone-like properties. Anethole is a chemical constituent within fennel and anise oil, which both have oestrogen-like properties, although its oestrogenic activity is many times weaker than that of oestrogen. Citral, another chemical constituent found in citrus fruits, may also have slight oestrogenic effects, but further research is needed in order to confirm this.

Essential oils with possible hormonal activity These plants may have possible hormonal activity: fennel, lemon grass, may chang and true melissa.

Caution: Owing to its oestrogen-like effect, fennel essential oil should not be used for people with oestrogen-dependent cancers (including breast cancer) or endometriosis, nor while pregnant or breast-feeding.

Pre-menstrual syndrome (PMS)

Symptoms and causes

Pre-menstrual syndrome is a combination of various physical and emotional symptoms that occur in some women for a week or two before menstruation. Emotional symptoms of PMS are irritability, tension, depression, fatigue and food cravings. Physical symptoms include breast tenderness, fluid retention, headache, backache and lower abdominal pain. It is generally thought to be caused by changes in hormone levels at this time of the menstrual cycle, but possible contributory factors are a poor diet, stress and overwork.

Recommended essential oils

Clary sage is a good tonic for the womb, regulating irregular periods and easing painful cramps in the lower abdomen. It combats excessive perspiration generally, and its euphoric properties lift depression and relieve tension and anxiety.

Geranium stimulates the adrenal cortex which in turn governs the balance of hormones. It can be used for pre-menstrual depression, lack of vaginal secretion and heavy periods and, with its diuretic properties, relieve inflammation and congestion of the breasts.

Rose otto is a stimulating tonic for the womb, calming and regulating. It is also warming and uplifting for the emotions, relieving stress and giving comfort.

Rose

Synergistic blend

✳ 2 drops clary sage
✳ 3 drops geranium
✳ 1 drop rose otto

Massage carrier base

✳ 15ml (½fl oz) sunflower oil
✳ 15 drops evening primrose oil

Methods of use

✳ Regular full body massage
✳ Massage abdomen daily one week before menstruation or onset of symptoms.
✳ Bathing
✳ Personal perfume

Other useful essential oils

Camomile (German and Roman), cypress, frankincense, grapefruit, juniper berry, lavender, neroli, sandalwood, vetiver and ylang ylang.

Herbal tradition

Clary sage's botanical name, *Salvia sclarea*, is derived from the Latin words for 'clear', 'saving' and 'healing'.

Geranium is native to South Africa, but is widely cultivated elsewhere. There are several oil-producing species, but *Pelargonium graveolens* is the one aromatherapists consider to be the best because of its delicate perfume.

Rose petals were once scattered by the Romans during the feast of Flora, the goddess of flowers. The rose is also associated with the Greek goddess of love, Aphrodite.

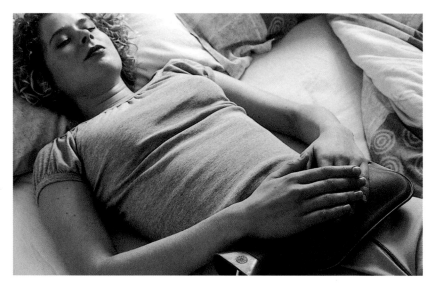

uterine problems. It releases painful cramps in the lower back by helping the muscles relax.

Jasmine relieves spasm in the uterus and soothes menstrual pain.

Synergistic blend
✳ 3 drops Roman camomile
✳ 2 drops clary sage
✳ 1 drop jasmine

Massage carrier base
✳ 10ml (⅙fl oz) sunflower oil

Methods of use
✳ Full body massage a couple of days before menstruation is due
✳ Warm compress
✳ Bathing
✳ During the period, massage the abdomen gently with the synergistic and carrier blend. Use a circular movement, and then place a warm heat pack on the abdomen. The heat pack will help the essential oils penetrate more quickly; this will relax the muscles and relieve the pain.

Herbal tradition
Camomile was considered to be a sacred herb by the ancient Egyptians, who dedicated it to their gods.

Clary sage was used during medieval times for digestive disorders, kidney disease and menstrual complaints.

Jasmine is a well-used oil and has long been associated in folklore with warming of the womb. It is used during labour and birth, as well as to treat menstrual problems.

Painful periods

Symptoms and causes
Painful periods, also known as dysmenorrhoea, are associated with the hormonal changes that occur during a period. They are typically felt as cramp-like pain or discomfort in the lower abdomen, which usually comes and goes. There may also be a dull ache in the lower back. Severe pain may be symptomatic of a gynaecological disorder which may need the attention of a specialist.

Recommended essential oils
Roman camomile helps regulate the menstrual cycle and eases period pain.

Clary sage is a good tonic for the womb and particularly helpful with

Other useful essential oils
Cypress, frankincense, juniper berry, lavender, sweet marjoram, true melissa and rose otto.

Menopause

Symptoms and causes

When women reach their menopause, physical and psychological changes take place in the body, caused by a reduction in the amount of oestrogen produced by the ovaries as they gradually wind down egg production. The term 'menopause' literally means cessation of menstruation, but is generally used to denote the transitional time before, during and after this specific point (which can only be determined retrospectively).

The symptoms of menopause can start as early as in the 30s, but usually affect women in their 40s and 50s. These may include hot flushes and night sweats, vaginal dryness, sleep disturbance, poor memory, poor concentration, tearfulness, anxiety, stress and loss of interest in sex. Severity of symptoms may also be related to stress and poor diet.

Other useful essential oils

Roman camomile, clary sage, frankincense, geranium, lavender, true melissa, neroli, rose otto, sandalwood and ylang ylang.

Recommended essential oils

Bergamot has a sedative yet uplifting character that is excellent for anxiety, depression and stress. It is a cleansing tonic for the uterus.

Cypress is excellent for excessive sweating, oedema and heavy menstruation. It has a calming effect on the mind, soothing anger and frustration.

Fennel is an excellent body cleanser and is said to activate the glandular system by imitating the hormone oestrogen. This makes it useful for menopausal problems such as irregular periods, pre-menstrual tension and low sexual response.

Synergistic blend
* 2 drops bergamot
* 2 drops cypress
* 2 drops fennel

Massage carrier base
* 15ml (½fl oz) sunflower oil
* 10 drops borage oil

Methods of use
* Regular full body massage
* Bathing
* Personal perfume

Herbal tradition

Cypress has a fresh, clean, pine-needle aroma, like most evergreen oils.

Fennel is an ancient herb used traditionally to give courage and strength, and has a sweet, aniseed-like aroma. It also has oestrogenic properties, which can help with problems such as obesity and water retention.

Muscles and bones

Our skeletal system is like a cage, resilient and strong, which enables us to walk upright and provides protection for our vital organs. The muscle structure comprises bundles of specialized cells, which are capable of contraction and relaxation to create movement of the skeletal structure via messages transmitted from the brain to the nervous system.

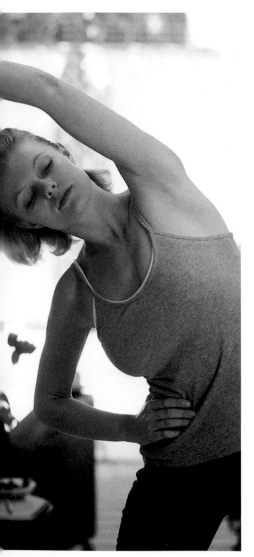

Muscles

Muscles cover the main framework of the skeleton of the body. These are responsible for 50 per cent of our bodyweight and their function is to permit movement. There are two types of muscle: voluntary and involuntary. The voluntary muscles, such as those used in walking or writing, are under conscious control. Involuntary muscles are those involved in movements of the heart, respiration, digestion and so on, and are outside conscious control.

All muscles work in antagonistic pairs and groups. As one set of muscle fibre contracts, its opposite set relaxes. Muscle movement produces waste such as carbon dioxide and lactic acid. A good flow of blood to the muscles helps remove this waste, which is eventually excreted via the urinary system, skin and lungs.

When overworked or distressed, muscles become sticky and congested. Aromatherapy can help to improve muscle tone by detoxifying the system and normalizing the acid/alkaline composition of the blood. Treatment is geared to reducing stress and increasing flexibility. This can be achieved by using a combination of methods: mineral salt baths, aromatherapy massage, compresses, gentle stretching, deep breathing and relaxation exercises.

Bones

The skeleton is a hard framework of 206 bones. Bones are living tissue made from special cells called osteoblasts. The tissue varies considerably in density and compactness: the closer to the surface of the bone, the more compact it is. Many bones have a central cavity containing marrow, a tissue that is the source of most of the cells of the blood and is also a site for the storage of fats. The functions of the bones are:

* to support the body and give it shape
* to enable movement
* to protect delicate body organs
* to produce blood cells in the red bone marrow
* to form joints, which are essential for the movement of the body
* to provide attachment for muscles, so that the body can be moved in different directions
* to provide a store of calcium salts and phosphorus

Arthritis and rheumatism

Symptoms and causes

There are many forms of arthritis and rheumatism, including bursitis, gout, sciatica, osteoarthritis and rheumatoid arthritis. Osteoarthritis is caused by natural wearing of the joints as the body ages, whereas rheumatoid arthritis is an aggressive disease leading to destruction of the joints. In all cases, movement of the joints can be painful and restricted, and they can also swell periodically. Some possible causes (other than specific diseases) of pain in the joints are heredity, chronic emotional depression, age-related wear and tear, food allergies, injury or over-use of muscles and joints.

Recommended essential oils

Celery seed has exceptional diuretic properties that help to dissolve accumulated lactic acid in the joints, clearing the body of toxins and purifying the blood. The effect on the mind is one of hope.

Frankincense helps with chronic emotional depression, releasing past anger and hurt. It is a forgiving oil that helps the person concerned come to terms with whatever problem they may have or had. Frankincense also helps to relax the body.

Handy hint
Take three 500mg capsules of evening primrose oil or borage oil daily.

Juniper berry helps to eliminate lactic acid and swelling, easing stiff movement and pain.

Synergistic blend
✳ 2 drops celery seed
✳ 1 drop frankincense
✳ 3 drops juniper berry

Massage carrier base
✳ 15ml (½fl oz) sunflower oil
✳ 15 drops hypericum oil
✳ 3 drops neem seed oil

Celery leaf and seed

Methods of use
✳ Regular full body massage
✳ Massage gently above (not directly on) painful joints
✳ Bath salts in bath
✳ Compress

Caution: Never apply massage over inflamed and swollen joints. Allow the swelling to go down before gently massaging the affected area.

Herbal tradition
Celery seed has traditionally been widely used for bladder and kidney complaints, digestive upsets and menstrual problems. It is quoted in the *British Herbal Pharmacopoeia* as a specific for rheumatoid arthritis with mental depression.

Other useful essential oils
Cajuput, Roman camomile, cedarwood (Atlas and Virginian), cypress, eucalyptus (*Eucalyptus globulus*), ginger, lavender, lemon, Spanish marjoram, sweet marjoram, niaouli, rosemary and sweet thyme.

Muscular aches and pains

Symptoms and causes

Muscular aches and pains are one of the most common reasons for people to visit their doctor. Generally, the causes range from pulled muscles, poor posture and repetitive movement to over-exertion. The pain, if caused by a recent injury, will be sharp. For old injuries and muscular tension, the pain is usually a dull ache. Stiffness and cramp may also occur in the joints.

Rosemary

Herbal tradition
Peppermint has been cultivated since ancient times in China and Japan. In Egypt, evidence of peppermint has been found in tombs dating from 1000 BCE.

Rosemary has been held as sacred in many civilizations, and is symbolic of remembrance and loyalty. The Greeks dedicated it to Apollo, god of medicine, music, poetry and prophesy. In medieval times, garlands or sprigs of rosemary were worn for good luck.

Other useful essential oils
Angelica, basil, bergamot, cajuput, clove, coriander, eucalyptus (*Eucalyptus globulus*), fennel, ginger, juniper berry, sweet marjoram, Spanish marjoram, lavender (one that originated in eastern Europe) and sweet thyme.

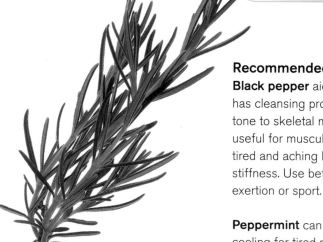

Recommended essential oils
Black pepper aids circulation and has cleansing properties that give tone to skeletal muscles, making it useful for muscular aches and pains, tired and aching limbs and muscular stiffness. Use before excessive exertion or sport.

Peppermint can be warming or cooling for tired muscles, and helps general numbness in the limbs.

Rosemary is a stimulating, pain-relieving agent, which helps dissolve lactic acid and ease tired, overworked muscles.

Synergistic blend
* 2 drops black pepper
* 2 drops peppermint
* 2 drops rosemary

Massage carrier base
* 15ml (½fl oz) sunflower oil
* 15 drops hypericum oil
* 3 drops neem seed oil

Methods of use
* Regular full body massage
* Massage gently above (not directly on) painful joints
* Bath salts in bath
* Compress

Caution: Never massage if the muscle is inflamed and swollen. Use a cold compress instead.

Back pain

Symptoms and causes

Many things can cause back pain. Discomfort in a certain region can range from a dull ache to a sharp pain. It can be localized to one area, or can spread to other regions, such as the leg. Movements can intensify the pain or indeed improve it. Muscle strains are a common occurrence, and result in acute and severe pain when the sufferer attempts to carry out certain movements, such as bending forward, turning over while lying down or attempting to get into and out of a car.

Lumbago is synonymous with chronic back pain; this is a dull ache across the lower regions of the back. There is no apparent cause; however, the most likely factor is the formation of nodules and fibrous congestion, which impinge on nearby nerves. If the pain radiates down the back of the legs behind the knees then the cause of your back pain could be sciatica, in which the vertebrae of the spine misalign and inflame or trap a nerve root.

Recommended essential oils

Bay helps nerve-end pain and has a warming effect where there is coldness within the muscles.

Clove has pain-relieving properties affecting the nerve end pathways that can help with localized pain.

Lemon is a superb tonic to the circulatory system, cleansing the body of waste, and works well with neuralgic pain.

Synergistic blend
* 2 drops bay
* 1 drop clove
* 2 drops lemon

Massage carrier base
* 15ml (½fl oz) sunflower oil
* 15 drops hypericum oil

Methods of use
* Regular full body massage
* Gentle massage over painful area
* Bath salts in the bath
* Compress

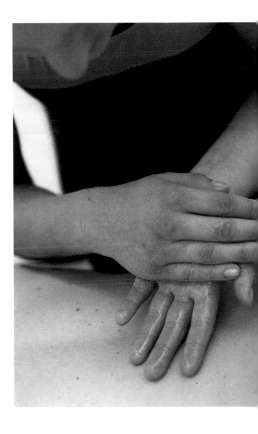

Other useful essential oils
Cajuput, Roman camomile, eucalyptus (*Eucalyptus globulus*), ginger, lavandin, lavender, sweet marjoram, peppermint and rosemary.

Handy hint
With lower back problems, deep thumb stroking in a circular movement over the whole of the lower back and bottom will help increase the circulation of the lumbar muscles, thereby reducing the tightness and knotted areas. This will help break up fibrous congestion, clear oedema and ease pain in the lower back.

Skin care

The skin that covers the body (see structure diagram on page 17) is a sensitive organ and, just like other vital parts of the body, it responds to our diet, lifestyle and emotions. If we are under stress, it can become dry and taut, and in severe emotional states – such as bereavement – it may even become seriously dehydrated. Hormonal changes can produce spots and blemishes. Cigarette smoke and pollution can age skin by making it grey and causing premature wrinkles and lines.

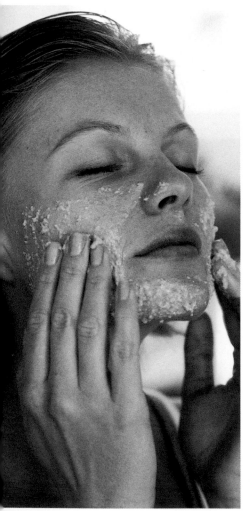

Aromatherapy, in conjunction with other treatments such as exfoliation or skin brushing, can help keep skin supple and young-looking. Regular treatments such as these will thoroughly ceanse the skin and replace lost nutrients and moisture.

Daily routine

The following daily routine is suitable for all skin types.

✳ Wash your face twice a day with a mild, pH-balanced cleansing bar. This helps balance the skin's acid mantle, which is a mixture of sebum and fluid that supports the skin's defence against infection.

✳ After washing, tone your face with pure floral water, using camomile for greasy skin, rose for sensitive skin and lavender for healing. Floral waters are produced from the distillation of the plant. They will make your skin feel clean, fresh and invigorated.

✳ Moisturize the skin with a combination of beeswax, coconut oil and essential oils, or with a light-textured vegetable oil such as apricot kernel, peach kernel or jojoba (see the Directory of carrier oils, pages 124–125). Do not use mineral oils, because they clog the skin and contribute to pimples, spots and blackheads.

Steam cleansing

Once a week, the skin of the face, especially congested or oily skin that is prone to spots and blackheads, will benefit from the deep cleansing effect of an aromatic facial sauna or steaming with a towel, which have the following effects:

✳ Opening of the follicles, allowing a deeper cleansing of dirt, grease and blackheads.

✳ Softening of dead surface cells, which aids in their removal when cleansing.

✳ Aiding the sweat glands to rid themselves of toxins.

✳ Increasing the circulation of the blood to the face so that the tissues are nourished. This leaves the skin feeling soft and gives a healthy glow to the complexion.

Facial saunas

Steam clean your face with essential oils once a week, either by filling a bowl with warm water and placing a towel over your head to trap the steam, or by using an electric facial steamer. Always finish the treatment by splashing your face with cold water to tone and refresh the skin.

Towel steaming

Place a synergistic blend of essential oils in a bowl of warm water, submerge the towel and wring it out thoroughly. Drape the towel over your face and relax. The towel should remain on your face for approximately two minutes. If required, repeat the procedure. After towel steaming, always cleanse and tone the face.

Caution: Avoid facial saunas and towel steaming if you suffer from asthma, since the steam may trigger an attack.

Clay face packs or masks

Face masks are beneficial for all types of skin. They can nourish, stimulate, cleanse and exfoliate the outer skin layer. Other benefits are that they can soothe and calm inflammation, clear impurities and act as an anti-wrinkle treatment. In all

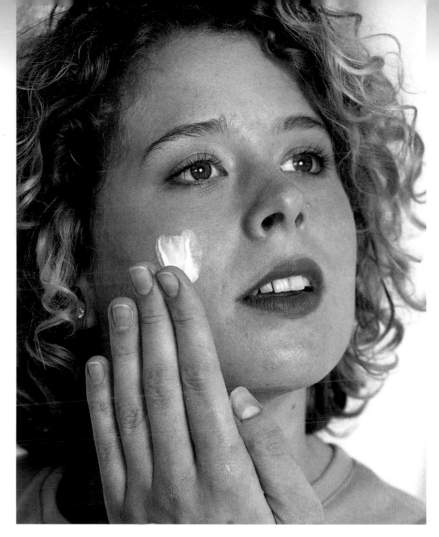

cases, a face mask improves the colour and tone of a face.

Clays are natural products, which have absorbed the plant and minerals of the earth over many years. There are red, yellow, green, white, black and brown clays. Some of these are very drying for the skin, so it is best to use green clay, which can be used for all kinds of skin conditions. Green clay is useful for treating acne and inflamed skin, but is gentle enough for mature skin. It can be used to balance combination skin, normalize oily skin and revitalize dry skin. Its antiseptic action will act as an

emollient, which leaves the skin feeling silky smooth. The stimulating effect of the clay will increase the lymph flow and circulation, which enables oxygen to speed the elimination of waste products. It is rich in calcium, magnesium, potassium and sodium.

Make a synergy of essential oils. Take 1 drop from the synergy, and add it to 1 teaspoon of powered green clay and 1 teaspoon of floral water. Apply the mixture to clean skin, avoiding the delicate eye area, and leave on for ten minutes. Rinse off in warm, then cool, water.

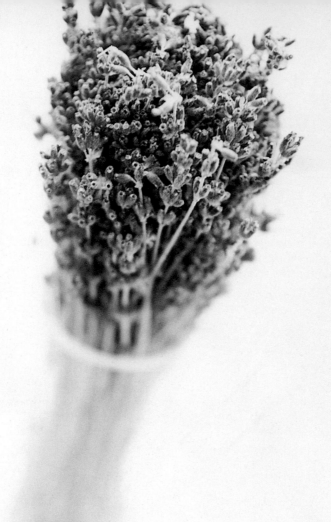
Lavender

Facial carrier base
✳ 20ml (¾fl oz) apricot kernel or peach kernel oil
✳ 15 drops jojoba oil
✳ 5 drops camellia oil

Methods of use
✳ Facial steam cleansing
✳ Clay face pack once a week

Other useful essential oils
Angelica, German camomile, frankincense, jasmine and palmarosa.

Handy hint
Add 2 drops of the synergistic blend and 1 level teaspoon of bicarbonate of soda to a small bowl of warm water. Soak strips of cotton wool in the water and place on the oily 'T' zone of the face. This will bring out the impurities along the greasy 'T' zone but not dry out the areas of the face that are already dry.

Combination skin

Characteristics
The chin, nose and forehead form an oily 'T' zone on the face. The skin around the eyes, cheeks and neck can be dry.

Recommended essential oils
Geranium is useful for all skin types, because it balances the sebum, which is the fatty secretion in sebaceous glands that keeps the skin supple.

Lavender is valuable for all skin conditions, because it promotes growth of new cells and exerts a balancing action on sebum.

Ylang ylang is a versatile oil that has a balancing action on sebum. This means it is effective on both oily and dry skins.

Synergistic blend
✳ 1 drop geranium
✳ 2 drops lavender
✳ 1 drop ylang ylang

Mature skin

Characteristics

As skin ages, it becomes less elastic, and lines and wrinkles may start to appear. Essential oils are excellent for helping to preserve the youthful appearance of the skin, and for rejuvenating mature skin, since certain essential oils help the regeneration of new skin cells.

Recommended essential oils

Carrot seed improves the complexion, due to its strengthening effect on red blood cells, adding tone and elasticity to the skin. It gives a youthful appearance and is said to remove 'liver' spots from the skin.

Frankincense gives a lift to ageing skin and is cell-rejuvenating.

Galbanum softens mature skin.

Synergistic blend
* 1 drop carrot seed
* 1 drop frankincense
* 1 drop galbanum

Facial carrier base
* 20ml (¾fl oz) apricot kernel or peach kernel oil
* 15 drops carrot oil
* 5 drops rose hip oil

Methods of use
* Facial steam cleansing
* Clay face pack once a week

Recipe for clay face pack for mature skin
* 5g (¼oz) green clay
* 5 drops apricot kernel or peach kernel oil
* 2 drops carrot oil
* 1 drop rose hip oil
* 1 drop synergistic blend essential oils

Other useful essential oils
Rose otto and sandalwood.

Other useful carrier oils
Avocado, borage, camellia and macadamia.

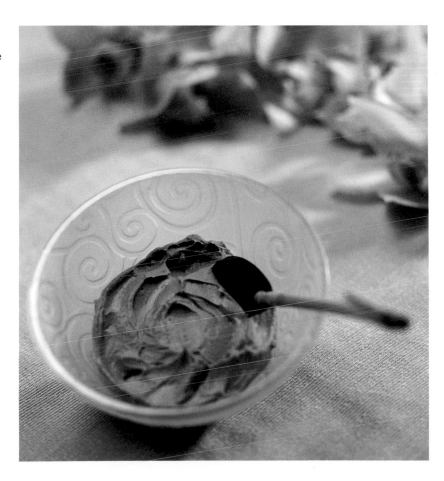

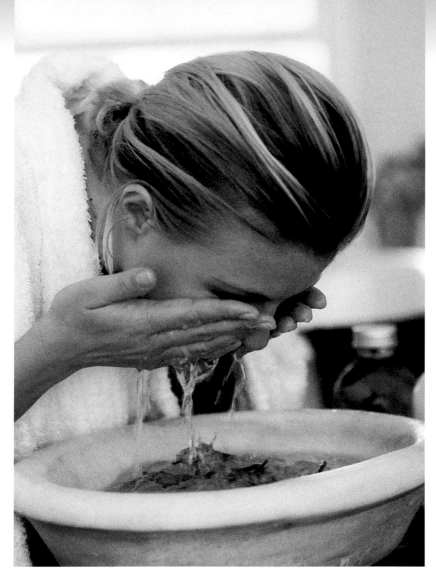

Recommended essential oils

Jasmine is a highly effective balm and tonic for dry and sensitive skin.

Lavender is a valuable balancing oil for all skin conditions.

Mandarin is a gentle oil that is excellent for sensitive skins.

Synergistic blend
✳ 1 drop jasmine
✳ 2 drops lavender
✳ 1 drop mandarin

Facial carrier base
✳ 20ml (¾fl oz) sunflower oil
✳ 15 drops carrot oil
✳ 5 drops evening primrose oil

Methods of use
✳ Facial steam cleansing
✳ Clay face pack once a week

Sensitive skin

Characteristics

People with sensitive skin need to avoid products that contain synthetic ingredients, such as perfume, lanolin, mineral oil and sometimes soap. There are two main types of skin sensitivity. The first one is contact allergic dermatitis, which consists of red, itchy patches, that may blister. The patches will correspond to the area where the substance was applied, and will develop between a few hours or two days after contact. The second type of sensitivity is contact urticaria, which causes red, itchy, raised areas on the skin. This can develop within a few minutes to half an hour after skin contact with some medications, chemicals, plants, insect bites and foods. A person with sensitive skin may have oily skin or dry skin and should choose products suitable for that skin type, ensuring that they are pure and natural.

Other useful essential oils
Geranium, true melissa, neroli, palmarosa, rose otto and sandalwood.

Other useful carrier oils
Camellia and jojoba.

Dry skin

Characteristics

Dry skin is a common problem, and can actually be caused by a lack of fluid intake. Other causes are lost moisture and insufficient oil production. An effective moisturizer will replace the moisture lost, while essential oils will normalize the production of natural oil.

Recommended essential oils

Benzoin is particularly good for cracked and dry skin, making it more elastic.

Patchouli is excellent for dry skin because it promotes regrowth of skin cells.

Sandalwood is generally a balancing oil that is especially good for dry, ageing and dehydrated skins.

Synergistic blend

✳ 1 drop benzoin
✳ 1 drop patchouli
✳ 1 drop sandalwood

Facial carrier base

✳ 20ml (¾fl oz) sweet almond oil
✳ 15 drops avocado oil
✳ 5 drops wheatgerm oil

Methods of use

✳ Facial steam cleansing
✳ Clay face pack once a week

Handy hint

Towel steam using 2 drops of the synergistic blend. This will soften the dead surface cells so that they can be removed easily when cleansing.

Other useful essential oils

German camomile, lavender, neroli and rose otto.

Other useful carrier oils

Borage, calendula, camellia, coconut, evening primrose, jojoba, rose hip and sunflower.

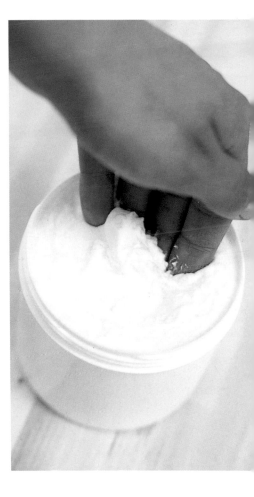

Oily skin

Characteristics

Excessive oiliness of the skin is caused by an overproduction of sebum in the tiny sebaceous glands just beneath the surface of the skin. Sebum is a natural lubricant, which everybody needs for the well-being and good appearance of their skin.

Too much sebum produces a greasy appearance, which is often associated with spots and blackheads. This is usually more marked in adolescence due to the fact that sebum production is linked to the activity of the whole endocrine system, which is in a stage of change following puberty. A long-term benefit of oily skin, however, is that it will age far more slowly than skin that is relatively dry.

Aromatherapy treatments can help to fight the bacteria which flourish on the surface of oily skin. They will also help to normalize and reduce the production of oil in the sebaceous glands.

Recommended essential oils

Juniper berry is a good tonic for oily and congested skin. Its purifying properties help to ease acne and blocked pores. It is important to note, however, that when using juniper berry oil the condition may get worse before it gets better as impurities are drawn out, but the result will be clearer, fresher skin.

Niaouli heals skin eruptions, boils and ulcers, and is useful for washing infected wounds.

Sweet orange is a good skin tonic that refreshes the skin and eliminates toxins from congested pores.

Synergistic blend

* 1 drop juniper berry
* 1 drop niaouli
* 2 drops sweet orange

Facial carrier base

* 20ml (¾fl oz) jojoba oil
* 20 drops hypericum oil

Methods of use

* Facial steam cleansing twice a week
* Clay face pack twice a week

Other useful essential oils

Bergamot, cedarwood (Atlas and Virginian), clary sage, cypress, geranium, lavender, lemon, lime, palmarosa, tea tree and vetiver.

✳

Other useful carrier oils

Macadamia and sunflower.

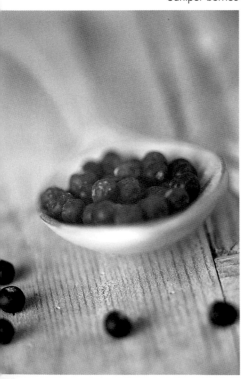

Juniper berries

Acne

Characteristics

There are four main causes of acne: hormonal imbalance, accumulations of toxins, stress and diet. All these factors should be addressed when treating acne. Essential oils in a skincare product help in a number of ways when applied to the problem area. They are antibacterial. They encourage circulation and therefore the removal of waste matter. They deep cleanse the skin and help return it to normal by balancing the secretions of the sebaceous glands.

Recommended essential oils

Basil is a revitalizing tonic that stimulates the skin, cleansing sluggish and congested pores and leaving the skin feeling refreshed.

Lemon grass is an effective oil for open pores, and it balances oily conditions.

Niaouli is a tissue-firming oil beneficial for cleansing skin eruptions associated with acne.

Synergistic blend

* 1 drop basil
* 1 drop lemon grass
* 1 drop niaouli

Facial carrier base

* 20ml (¾fl oz) jojoba oil
* 20 drops hypericum oil

Methods of use

* Facial steam cleansing
* Clay face pack once a week
* Massage. Use the following technique when applying the synergistic and carrier blends above. Start at the chin and gently squeeze a small section of the skin between the thumb and fingers, giving the skin a slight kneading movement. This helps to empty the oil ducts. Continue the movement up over the cheeks and over the forehead. The skin on the forehead may be too tight to twist; therefore, place the tips of the fingers parallel to one another and push gently towards each other.

Other useful essential oils
Cajuput, peppermint, tagetes and vetiver.

Other useful carrier oils
Calendula, carrot, evening primrose, grapeseed, sunflower and wheatgerm.

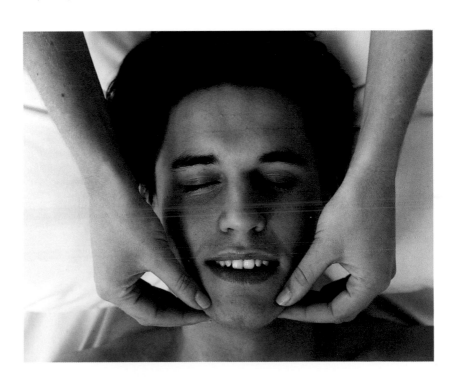

Head lice

What are head lice?

Head lice are small insects that thrive in hair – clean or dirty – and feed on the blood of the scalp. They are most commonly found in children. In most cases, the head is not 'crawling with lice' – often there are fewer than ten adult lice present. Full-grown lice are about 3mm (⅛in) in length and are not easily seen. Each can lay up to 300 eggs, or 'nits', which become attached to the base of the hair shaft. Development from hatching to adult takes 9–14 days. The lice do not fly or jump; they can only transfer from one head to another when two heads are in close proximity, or through shared use of combs or brushes.

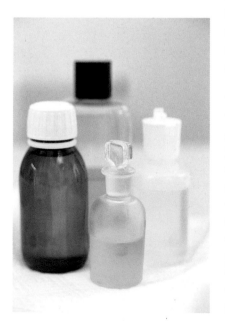

Although some people may experience itching, more often than not there are no obvious symptoms. The most likely site for eggs is behind the ears and at the nape of the neck. Live lice may be seen anywhere close to the scalp.

Combing

Checking the hair regularly, and combing wet hair with a 'detector' comb, are the best ways to check for live lice. Detector combs have fine teeth, so even very young lice cannot pass through them. Lice in dry hair move rapidly away from any disturbance, but stay still in wet hair.

When combing, make sure the hair is combed from the roots, with the teeth of the comb touching the scalp, to the tips. Always use the bug-buster conditioning blend (see right), to make combing easier. The comb should be wiped after each stroke with a white cloth.

Treatment regime

The bug-buster regime requires four conditioning/combing sessions at half-weekly intervals over a two-week period. The first session helps remove all the hatched lice. After the first session, any newly hatched lice will not move for a couple of days, so they cannot be passed on to other people. If full-grown lice are found in the second, third or fourth sessions, the head has been re-infected, and the regime must be started again. In each session, follow this procedure:

✳ Ensure that the eyes are well protected.

✳ Prepare the bug-buster conditioning blend (see below) and massage into the scalp.

✳ Leave the mixture on the head for half an hour, or up to two hours.

✳ A plastic cap will help absorption and stop children from touching the hair.

✳ Comb the hair.

✳ To remove the bug-buster blend, massage in neat shampoo initially, then rinse and shampoo as normal.

Bug-buster blend

Add the following essential and carrier oils to 50ml (2fl oz) of non-perfumed conditioner:

✳ For adults: 10 geranium, 10 drops lavender, 10 drops tea tree, 5 drops neem seed carrier oil.

✳ For children over 5 years: 3 drops geranium, 4 drops lavender, 3 drops tea tree, 2 drops neem seed carrier oil.

✳ For children aged 2–5: 1 drop geranium, 2 drops lavender, 2 drops tea tree, 1 drop neem carrier oil.

Caution: *Do not use on children under 2 years old.*

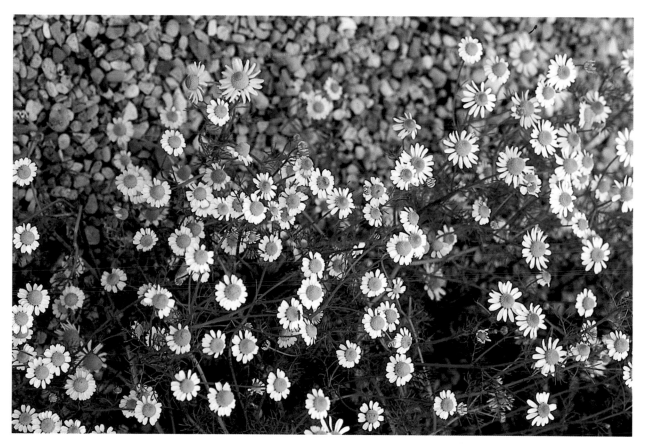

Roman camomile

Minor burns and abrasions

Caution: The advice given below is for minor burns and abrasions only. If you have a serious burn or wound, always seek medical advice before you use essential oils.

Burns and scalds

Superficial burns and scalds (first-degree burns) can be treated at home, because they involve only the outer layer of the skin. You will see a reddened, sometimes weepy area of skin, which will heal without leaving a permanent scar. First cool the affected area by placing it under running cold water, and then apply neat lavender oil. The lavender oil will take away the pain and promote rapid healing.

If you have a second- or third-degree burn, you should always seek medical advice.

Minor cuts and abrasions

Add 1 drop of Roman camomile, lavender or tea tree essential oil to water and wash the affected area with it. Cover with a clean lint and bandage.

Caution: Do not apply neat essential oils to wounds.

Emotions and mental energy

Aromatherapy is not just beneficial for physical ailments – it can also help with your emotions and your state of mind. Such conditions as nervous headaches, anxiety and stress (often one of the causes of a physical illness) can be eased by judicious use of the appropriate essential oils. Aromatherapy also helps promote a positive attitude to life, which is a vital aspect of overall good health and well-being.

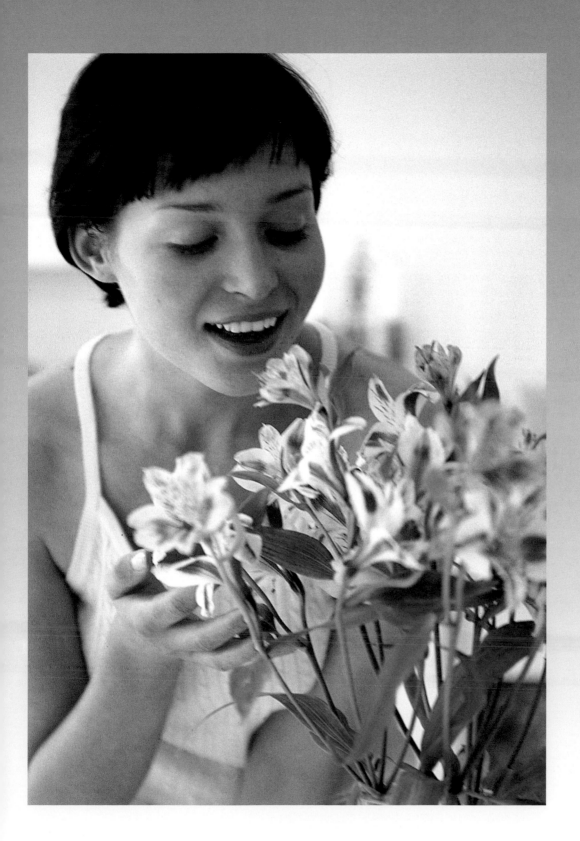

Balancing mind and body

It is now recognized that the chemicals in the brain form a continuous circuit not only with receptors in the brain but also with receptors in the immune system, the nervous system and the hormone system. It is impossible physiologically to separate the mind from the body. A strong constitution and a positive outlook on life together help to promote good health.

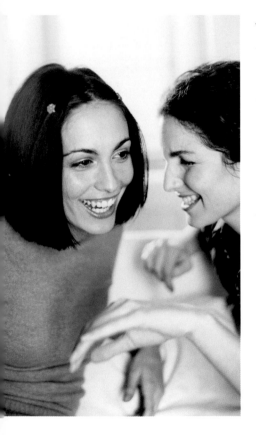

With a strong mental attitude, it is sometimes even possible for a person to cure disease in their own body. For example, stress and emotional factors are now recognized as important in the development of cancer. People have been known to cure themselves of cancer by addressing these aspects of their lives. Attitudes towards cancer have become more positive. Those who suffer are now encouraged to have a fighting spirit, and to do the things they have always wanted to do but never had the time. They are advised to meditate, to laugh, to think of putting themselves into a more positive frame of mind, to admit their problems, decide their priorities and, more importantly, to act upon them. This approach has produced some very good results.

The benefits of aromatherapy

Aromatherapy – the touch of the massage and the smell of the essential oils – is one of the finest treatments available for stress and the emotions. The properties of the essential oils release our inner feelings and open our minds. It is no accident that so many of the essential oils regarded as antidepressants are the product of summer flowers, for example, lavender, geranium, neroli, ylang ylang and rose. They evoke warm, sunny days and happy associations.

The touch of massage will ease tired muscles and, with a pleasing blend of your favourite oils, will be associated with feelings of relaxation. This helps to release tension, anxiety and stress, bringing a sense of calm and well-being.

Aromatherapy is a supportive therapy, which helps people cope with any type of illness. It is very useful for treating the physical symptoms of stress. Receiving smells and massage that promote relaxation helps the brain to maintain the body's balance so that organs can function efficiently. Make sure you choose essential oils that you like the smell of, otherwise you will not gain any benefits from them.

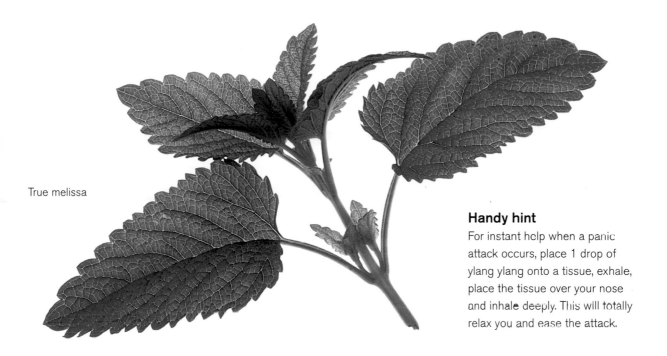

True melissa

Handy hint
For instant help when a panic attack occurs, place 1 drop of ylang ylang onto a tissue, exhale, place the tissue over your nose and inhale deeply. This will totally relax you and ease the attack.

Palpitations and panic attacks

Symptoms and causes
Palpitations or panic attacks can give you a rapid, forceful or irregular heartbeat. Possible causes are stress or over-use of stimulants such as caffeine or nicotine. They may be symptomatic of an underlying heart disorder, and, if recurrent, should be checked by a doctor.

Recommended essential oils
Lavender cleanses and soothes the spirit, relieving anger and exhaustion, resulting in a calmer approach to life.

True melissa has a calming yet uplifting effect on the emotions,

Herbal tradition
Melissa is one of the earliest recorded medicinal herbs. It was known as the 'elixir of life' and was used as a herbal remedy for the heart and emotions.

dealing with hypersensitive states. It is said to remove emotional blocks and is soothing in cases of panic and hysteria.

Rose otto has a soothing effect on the emotions, particularly depression, grief and bereavement. It lifts the heart and eases nervous tension and stress.

Synergistic blend
❋ 3 drops lavender
❋ 1 drop true melissa
❋ 2 drops rose otto

Massage carrier base
❋ 15ml (½fl oz) sweet almond oil

Methods of use
❋ Regular full body massage
❋ Dry inhalation
❋ Vaporizing
❋ Bathing

Other useful essential oils
Neroli and ylang ylang.

Anxiety

Symptoms and causes

It is normal to feel a little anxious when encountering life's upsets, such as family or work problems. Sometimes this feeling is useful as it can help to motivate us in dealing with demanding situations. Knowing when anxiety is a normal response to something is very important. For example, it is normal to worry about a child if they are late returning home, but it is not normal to feel anxious every moment that the child is out of sight.

Anxiety only becomes a problem when it is excessive. This occurs when the response to a situation is out of proportion or when anxiety is experienced without there being any objective, external reason for it.

Abnormal anxiety can result in many physical symptoms, including muscle fatigue, digestive problems, headaches and migraines, allergies, insomnia and heart disease. It is also an influencing factor in many other serious illnesses.

Other useful essential oils

Basil, bergamot, clary sage, frankincense, grapefruit, lavender, true melissa, neroli, bitter orange, patchouli and rose otto.

Recommended essential oils

May chang is uplifting to the mind, creating a sunny, bright outlook.

Petitgrain calms anger and panic, soothing the emotions.

Ylang ylang calms adrenaline flow and relaxes the nervous system. It will ease feelings of anger, shock, panic and fear.

Synergistic blend

* 2 drops may chang
* 3 drops petitgrain
* 1 drop ylang ylang

Massage carrier base

* 15ml (½fl oz) sunflower oil

Handy hint

People who suffer from anxiety usually work to a very high standard of achievement. Learn to accept that no one is perfect. When things get on top of you, step back for a moment, and learn to laugh at yourself and the rest of the world. It does not matter what other people think, only what you think of yourself. Treat yourself to daily aromatic baths and visit a professional therapist for regular holistic treatments.

Methods of use

* Regular full body massage
* Dry inhalation when you feel the start of the attack
* Vaporizing
* Bathing

Herbal tradition

May chang comes from a small tree native to Asia that has spicy fruits, fragrant leaves and flowers. The essential oil is derived from the spicy fruit. The Chinese use the fruit for cooking, since it is very similar to lemon grass. It is said to have been used to treat cancerous tumours, but is now widely used as an ingredient in soaps, perfumes and deodorants because of its spicy, uplifting perfume.

Stress

Symptoms and causes

When we push ourselves too hard, the first sign of stress is fatigue. If we then continually work against our body's wishes to rest, we start to interfere with both our mental health and our physical well-being. By ignoring the first signs, other symptoms such as anxiety, depression, palpitations, panic attacks and muscular aches and pains start to occur. Eventually we reach the stage where we cannot cope with the continued excessive demands made upon us.

Recommended essential oils

Fennel gives strength and courage in distress.

Geranium acts as a tonic to the nervous system, quelling anxiety and depression.

Grapefruit has overall balancing, uplifting and reviving qualities that makes it invaluable in times of stress.

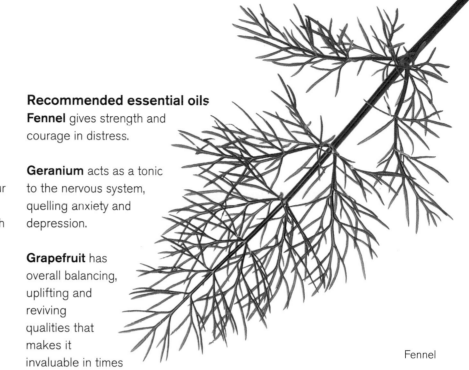

Fennel

Synergistic blend

✳ 1 drops fennel
✳ 3 drops geranium
✳ 2 drops grapefruit

Massage carrier base

✳ 15ml (½fl oz) sunflower oil

Methods of use

✳ Regular full body massage
✳ Vaporizing
✳ Bathing
✳ Own perfume
✳ Perfumed foam bath. Spend a few minutes each evening relaxing in your own perfumed foam bath. To 500ml (17fl oz) unscented foam bath, add 5 drops fennel, 15 drops geranium and 10 drops grapefruit and mix together in a blender. Put the blend in a plastic bottle. Squirt the mixture into the bath while the taps are running, to bring up the foam. Place scented candles around the room, turn off the lights and relax, inhaling the vapours deeply.

Herbal tradition

Geranium is thought to balance the mind and body because of its strong ability to regulate hormonal and emotional swings. There are over 700 varieties of cultivated geraniums, many of which are grown for ornamental purposes. The oil-producing species are *Pelargonium graveolens, P. odorantissimum* and *P. radens*.

Other useful essential oils

Basil, bay, bergamot, cardamom, cinnamon leaf, citronella, clary sage, frankincense, ginger, lavender, lemon grass, black pepper, peppermint, petitgrain, rose otto, rosemary and ylang ylang.

Headache and migraine

Symptoms and causes

There are many types of headache. Pain may be felt all over the head, or may occur in only one part. Sometimes the pain moves to another part of the head during the course of the headache. The pain can be throbbing, sharp, superficial or deep. Accompanying symptoms such as nausea and visual and sensory disturbances can also occur.

Possible causes are stress, tension and poor posture, which can cause tightening of the muscles in the face, neck and scalp. Other factors that may cause pain are hangovers, irregular meals, excessive sleep, sinusitis, toothache and head injury. Food additives, chocolate, cheese and red wine can cause a reaction in certain people.

Recommended essential oils

Bay has a warming and mildly analgesic effect on the emotions.

Sweet marjoram has pain-relieving and muscle-relaxing properties. It is also known to dilate the capillaries, allowing easier flow of blood, making it an exceptional oil for headaches and migraines.

Peppermint has a cooling and pain-relieving action that eases headaches and migraines.

Synergistic blend

* 2 drops bay
* 2 drops sweet marjoram
* 2 drops peppermint

Other useful essential oils

Roman camomile, clary sage, eucalyptus (*Eucalyptus globulus, E. smithii*), lavender and rosemary.

Herbal tradition

Marjoram's botanical name *Origanum* is derived from the Greek words *oros* and *ganos*, meaning 'joy of the mountains'. It lives up to this name, being fresh, warm and herbaceous with a slightly woody aroma.

Facial carrier base

* 15ml (½fl oz) sunflower oil

Methods of use

* Regular full body massage
* Massage the back of the neck. Make up the synergistic and carrier blend above, and using the tips of your fingers, make circular movements from the back of the neck upwards into the hairline. If you suffer regularly from migraine or headaches, do this every morning and night.
* Dry inhalation when you feel the start of the attack
* Steam inhalation to clear the head
* Bathing

Marjoram

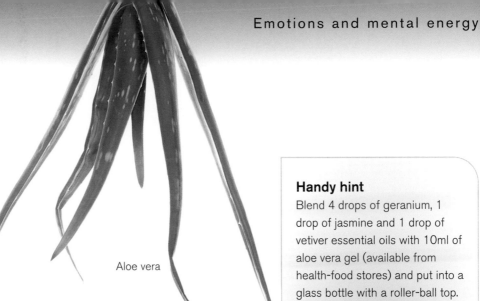

Aloe vera

Depression

Symptoms and causes

Depression involves feelings of sadness, hopelessness, pessimism and a general loss of interest in life, combined with a sense of reduced emotional well-being. It is natural to feel like this after a particularly sad event, such as the death of a loved one or the break-up of a relationship, but it becomes chronic when the feelings persist over a long period of time and refuse to disappear. There is no single obvious cause. Viral infections, hormonal disorders, stress, postnatal depression, heredity or lifestyle may trigger it.

Recommended essential oils

Immortelle seems to lessen the effects of fears and phobias, and helps relieve depression.

Herbal tradition

Sandalwood was used by yogis to encourage a contemplative state and enhance meditation. The Chinese use it to anoint and embalm the dead.

Rose otto has a soothing effect on the emotions, particularly sadness and grief cause by bereavement. It lifts the heart and gives a positive feeling of tender, loving care.

Sandalwood brings peace and quiet to a troubled mind, dealing with obsessional attitudes.

Synergistic blend
* 2 drops verbena
* 1 drop rose otto
* 1 drop sandalwood

Massage carrier base
* 15ml (½fl oz) sunflower oil

Methods of use
* Regular full body massage
* Vaporizing
* Bathing
* Own perfume

Caution: The above treatment is recommended only for cases of temporary, mild depression. If you suffer from chronic depression, seek professional help from a doctor or counsellor.

Handy hint

Blend 4 drops of geranium, 1 drop of jasmine and 1 drop of vetiver essential oils with 10ml of aloe vera gel (available from health-food stores) and put into a glass bottle with a roller-ball top. When you blend the essential oils with the gel, it will go cloudy; this is normal. Keep the bottle with you, and when you are feeling low, take it out and rub some of the gel on the inside of your wrists and behind your knees. This will give your spirits a positive lift. Aloe vera comes from the leaf of the cactus of this name, and is a healing agent for cuts, inflammations and burns. The gel is also very cooling.

Other useful essential oils

Basil, bergamot, cardamom, cinnamon, citronella, clary sage, coriander, fennel, frankincense, geranium, ginger, grapefruit, jasmine, lavender, lemon, lemon grass, orange (bitter and sweet), black pepper, peppermint, petitgrain, pine, rosemary, vetiver and ylang ylang.

Insomnia

Symptoms and causes

Insomnia is difficulty in falling asleep or in staying asleep. Sufferers may also experience daytime fatigue, irritability and difficulty in coping with everyday life. Possible causes of insomnia are worries about day-to-day living, or a difficult task. Stress, anxiety and depression can all cause an irregular sleep pattern.

Recommended essential oils

Grapefruit has an overall uplifting but calming quality, making it valuable in states of stress and worry.

Lavender has calming and sedative properties that give effective relief from insomnia.

Vetiver has a balancing effect on the central nervous system, instilling a more centred feeling. It is a calming oil for a busy mind, and will help with mental and physical exhaustion.

Synergistic blend

✻ 2 drops grapefruit
✻ 3 drops lavender
✻ 1 drop vetiver

Massage carrier base

✻ 15ml (½fl oz) sunflower oil

Methods of use

✻ Regular full body massage
✻ One or two drops of the synergistic blend on your pillow
✻ Vaporizing
✻ Bathing
✻ Own perfume

Herbal tradition

Grapefruit has the ability to overcome 'heavy' emotions that can weigh you down. It is high in vitamin C and is a valuable protection against infectious illness.

Lavender can act as a calming tonic for the nervous system, gently easing away stresses. The name 'lavender' comes from the Latin *lavare*, meaning 'to wash', since the Romans used to bathe in lavender-scented water.

Handy hint

Make or buy a herbal pillow. This will help soothe you to sleep while you inhale the aromas released when you put your head on the pillow.

Other useful essential oils

Benzoin, bergamot, camomile (German and Roman), Atlas cedarwood, celery seed, clary sage, frankincense, jasmine, mandarin, sweet marjoram, true melissa, neroli, petitgrain, rose otto, sandalwood, valerian and ylang ylang.

Lavender

Lack of concentration

Characteristics

Sometimes it is hard to focus on a particular thing. The mind is constantly distracted by irrelevant thoughts when it should be concentrating on the matter in hand, such as studying for an exam or gathering information for a new project. Essential oils can be very helpful in such situations. Research has shown that some odours, such as basil, cardamom, black pepper and rosemary, enhance the metabolic activity in the brain, increasing alertness.

Recommended essential oils

Basil sharpens the senses and encourages concentration.

Black pepper is very stimulating, strengthens the mind and gives stamina where there is frustration.

Peppermint is excellent for mental fatigue.

Synergistic blend

✳ 3 drops basil
✳ 3 drops black pepper
✳ 3 drops peppermint

Other useful essential oils

Bergamot, cardamom, lemon grass, may chang, bitter orange and rosemary.

Caution: This blend of essential oils will keep you awake at night.

Methods of use

✳ Vaporizing the synergistic blend
✳ If you do not have an electric diffuser or vaporizer, sprinkle the oils onto a tissue and place it behind a radiator. The heat from the radiator will diffuse the oils into the air.

Herbal tradition

Basil has a clean, uplifting aroma, which is fresh, pungent and reviving. In medieval times, it was believed that scorpions would breed under pots of basil, and just to smell the scent of basil would form a scorpion in the brain.

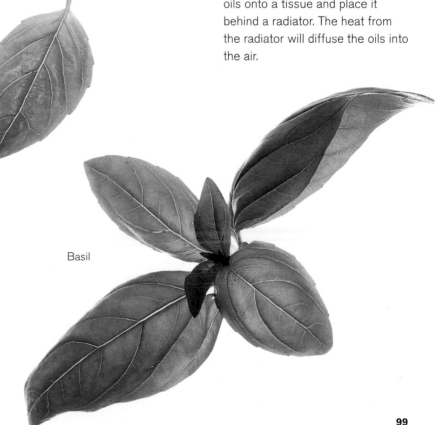

Basil

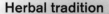

Memory loss

Characteristics

How often have you walked into a room to do something and forgotten what it was? Or maybe you find it difficult to recall facts and figures. This is a common experience. Forgetfulness affects children and adults alike, so there is no need to panic. Possible causes are lapses in concentration due to having too much on your mind. The brain is like a computer, with each compartment working separately. When you overload the memory compartment, it can become confused.

Recommended essential oils

Lemon is refreshing and helps to produce clarity of thought.

Rosemary energizes the brain cells and clears the head.

Sweet thyme strengthens the nerves and activates the brain cells, thereby aiding memory and concentration.

Synergistic blend

* 3 drops lemon
* 3 drops rosemary
* 3 drops sweet thyme

Method of use

* Vaporizing

Herbal tradition

Rosemary is fresh, invigorating and herbaceous, and can help to restore the senses. It can fight fatigue and debility, and revive a depressed spirit.

Handy hint

If you are studying for an exam, vaporize your study room with the synergistic blend in a diffuser. When you sit the exam, sprinkle the synergistic blend onto a tissue and take it with you. Smell the mix on the tissue during the exam and the essential oils will help you to remember vital pieces of information.

Other useful essential oils

Basil, bergamot, grapefruit, bitter orange, black pepper and peppermint.

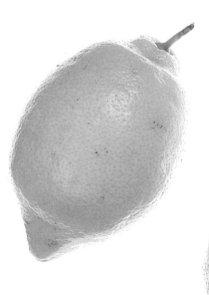

Lemon

Aphrodisiac perfumes

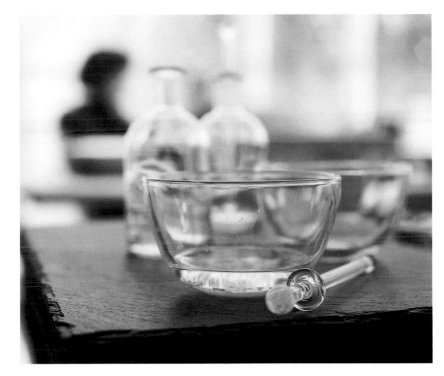

1 Synergistic blend: 3 drops bergamot, 2 drops sweet orange, 1 drop sandalwood.
Base: jasmine floral water.

2 Synergistic blend: 2 drops clary sage, 3 drops lavender, 1 drop patchouli.
Base: rose floral water.

3 Synergistic blend: 2 drops lemon, 2 drops petitgrain, 3 drops rosemary.
Base: neroli floral water.

Oil-based perfumes

Combine the following synergistic blends with 10ml jojoba carrier base oil, and put the mixture into a 10ml dark glass bottle. Apply the perfume to the pulse points, or warming zones, of the body; these are behind the ears, the sides of the neck, the inside of the wrists, the elbow creases, behind the knees and around the ankles. The warmth of the pulse points will release the perfume.

1 Synergistic blend: 2 drops coriander, 1 drop jasmine, 5 drops lemon.

2 Synergistic blend: 4 drops lavender, 2 drops bitter orange, 2 drops ylang ylang.

3 Synergistic blend: 4 drops clary sage, 2 drops frankincense, 2 drops grapefruit.

An aphrodisiac perfume is not just worn as a means of attraction, but should also enhance the mood of the wearer. Both partners must be open and receptive to the sensual perfume of the blend. Remember it is important that you both enjoy the smells you are creating, so when you blend these perfumes, have your partner in mind as well as yourself so that you create an essence that you can both enjoy. Aphrodisiac perfumes will not work on their own, but they will increase awareness of erotic sensations and enjoyable surroundings and of course, the company of your lover.

Easy ways to make a perfume

Aromatic floral waters

Distilled floral waters with essential oils added make an excellent perfume base, which can be sprayed onto the body or the hair, or around a room. Combine the following synergistic blends with the relevant floral water base, and put the mixture into a 50ml (2fl oz) bottle with an atomizer. When essential oils are added to water they will remain on top of the water so remember to shake the bottle before use.

Room-by-room guide to oils

Your home is a reflection of yourself and your family. It reflects your mood and the way you feel and live. The aroma in your home is very important; it can be creative and complement the colours and the style of your home. It will influence visitors' perception of who you are. When people walk into a house they immediately feel the atmosphere that surrounds it. How often do you feel when you enter somewhere new that the atmosphere is warm and inviting, without really knowing why? So, when you design and create your home environment, be aware of colour, smell and atmosphere. Decide what you want to portray and what you want other people to find out about you, because they will know you by your home.

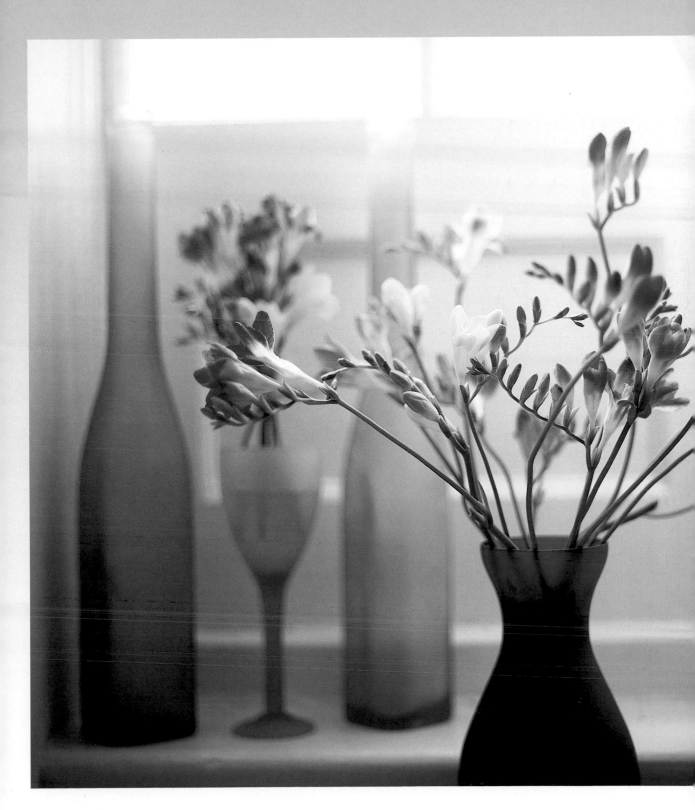

Hall

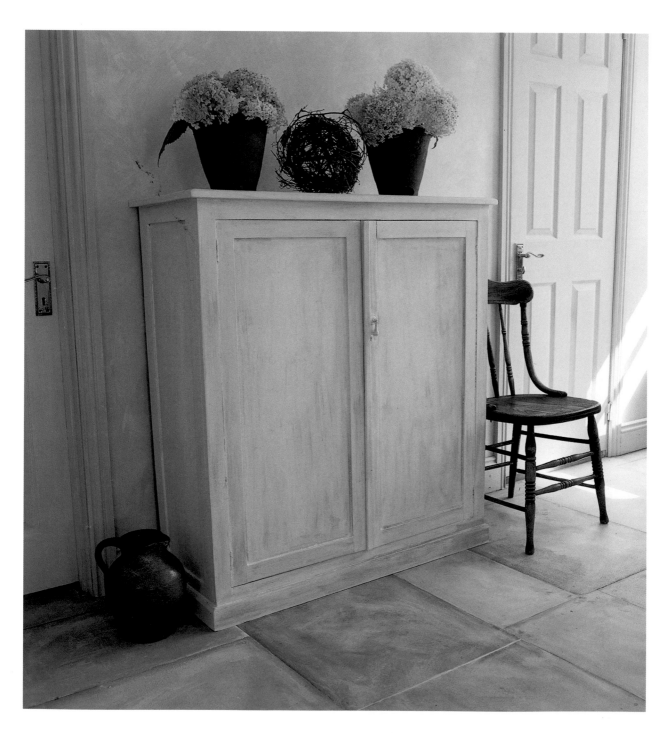

Often, when people think of a hall, they just regard it as the entrance to the house. It is easy to forget that this is the first impression people have of your lives. A dark, dreary hall, without any furniture, containing just the carpet and maybe the stairs leading to other levels, gives a feeling of coldness and lack of spirit within the home. A hall should welcome people in. This can be achieved by using warm, bright colours and materials in combination with essential oils. When the front door is opened in the middle of winter, when it may be cold and wet outside, visitors are immediately welcomed with a feeling of sunshine and the smell of refreshing citrus fruits.

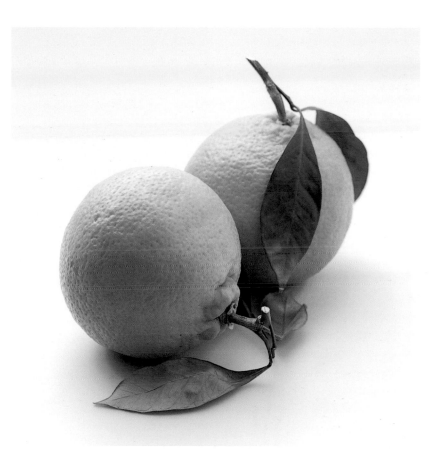

Recommended essential oils

The combination of these essential oils is light and airy, but they also have deodorizing and antiseptic qualities – a good combination for the hall: lemon, lime and bitter orange.

Infusion blend for fabrics and woods

First infuse ten small cottonwool balls with 10 drops each of lemon, lime and bitter orange essential oils. Then place the cottonwool balls in a large plastic bag together with any articles you wish to infuse, and leave them overnight. You will need to repeat this process every month to ensure the smell stays contained.

Room spray

Mix 3 drops each of lemon, lime and bitter orange essential oils into 300ml (10fl oz) of orange blossom floral water and put the mixture into a plant mist-sprayer with a very fine filter. Spray the room every evening before going to bed and close the doors. Tiny droplets of oil will settle on the carpet, enabling the oils to penetrate and stay in the room giving a lasting feeling of freshness and light.

Caution: When using essential oils in a room spray, avoid spraying wood, velvet and silk, because water stains may occur.

Kitchen

The kitchen produces many smells of its own from cooking, baking, pets, laundry and sometimes rotting vegetables. We do not want to mask the smells of the kitchen but can use the essential oils in a lot of ways by cleaning and deodorizing the air as well as the surfaces.

Recommended oils

All these essential oils will provide a clean, refreshing aroma for the kitchen and they also have bactericidal properties: citronella, elemi, lemon grass, lime, palmarosa and tea tree. Other useful essential oils are: grapefruit, mandarin, peppermint, pine and sweet thyme.

Methods of use

Room spray
In a plant mist-sprayer, mix 3 drops each of lemon grass, palmarosa and tea tree essential oils in 300ml (10fl oz) water. Spray into the air.

Insect-repellent
During the summer months when flies are a problem, use a vaporizing diffuser infused with 4 drops of citronella, 4 drops of lemon grass and 4 drops of peppermint. This is a very effective insect-repellent.

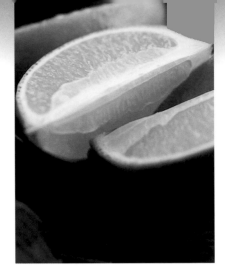

Cleaning the refrigerator or freezer
Add 1 drop each of lemon, tea tree and sweet thyme to the final rinse water, or alternatively drop the essential oils onto a kitchen towel and wipe over the surface when soaking up residual water. Using essential oils in this way for your appliances will work as an antiseptic and prevent fungal growth within the crevices. The subtlety of the oils means that there will not be an overpowering smell when you refill the refrigerator or freezer with food.

Synergistic blend for washing down kitchen surfaces
Mix together the following ingredients, and keep the synergistic blend in a dark glass bottle ready for use. When washing down work surfaces, cupboards, sinks, tiles, paintwork or the kitchen floor, add 6 drops to any environmentally friendly cleaning detergents.

※ 12 drops lemon
※ 30 drops palmarosa
※ 6 drops pine
※ 12 drops sweet thyme

Washing-up liquid
You can make up a washing-up liquid that is both environmentally friendly and delicious-smelling. Add 5 drops of grapefruit, 5 drops of lemon, 5 drops of lime and 10 drops of mandarin to a 500ml (17fl oz) bottle of a washing-up liquid that contains a vegetable detergent based on coconut oil. The natural aroma of the essential oils has uplifting properties, making washing-up less of a chore!

Washing and drying clothes
When washing clothes by machine, add 3–5 drops of your chosen essential oil to an unscented fabric conditioner.

When tumble-drying clothes, place 3–5 drops of an essential oil onto a small cotton handkerchief and pop it into the dryer with the rest of the clothes. For freshness, use geranium, grapefruit or lavender.

If clothes smell strongly of cigarettes or any other unpleasant odour, use clary sage, cypress and pine in the washing machine and tumble dryer.

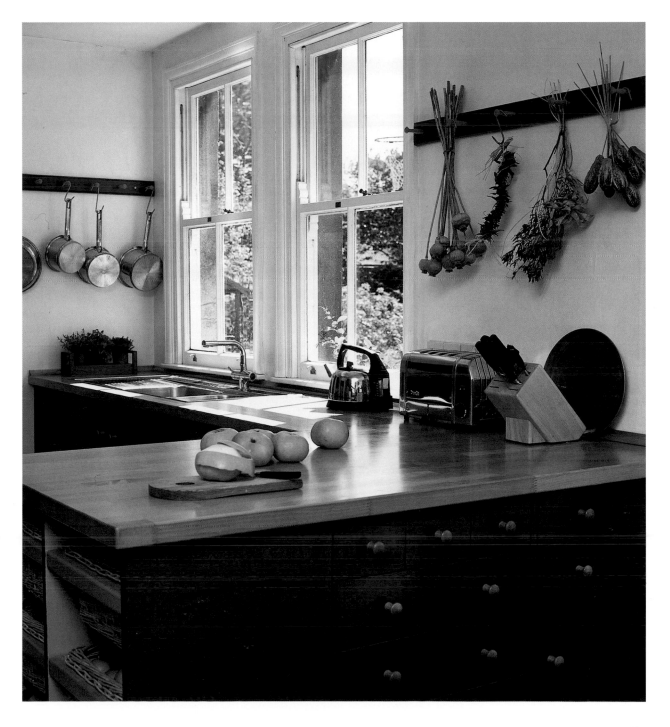

Dining room

The dining room, if you are lucky enough to have a separate one, is usually used for family eating and for entertaining friends. By using smell together with visual items, you can make it memorable for all those who eat there. Many annual events, theme dinners and parties may be enhanced by using essential oils to set the scene. Connecting a particular smell with a particularly happy occasion can provide a long-lasting and delightful memory.

Recommended essential oils

Your choice will depend upon the occasion and your mood. See the recommendations given below.

Methods of use

Themed meals
Try the following blends for diffusing essential oils for that special meal.

✳ Oriental: 5 drops ginger, 2 drops jasmine, 5 drops lemon grass.

✳ Indian: 1 drop cinnamon leaf, 3 drops coriander, 3 drops ginger, 5 drops bitter orange.

✳ Family meal: 2 drops basil, 4 drops geranium, 6 drops rosemary.

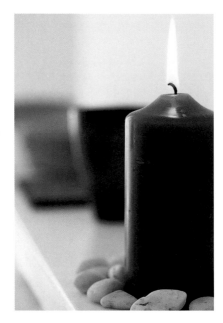

Blends for special occasions

✳ Children's birthday party: 2 drops cedarwood (Atlas or Virginian), 6 drops juniper, 4 drops lemon.

✳ Christmas: 2 drops cinnamon , 2 drops clove, 4 drops mandarin, 5 drops bitter orange.

✳ St Valentine's Day: 4 drops bergamot, 5 drops geranium, 1 drop jasmine, 2 drops rose.

✳ Easter: 6 drops frankincense, 5 drops grapefruit, 1 drop patchouli.

✳ Halloween: 2 drops cinnamon leaf, 4 drops bitter orange, 6 drops petitgrain.

Fragrant candles
Candle-making has become very popular, and it is relatively easy to do with the advent of candle kits. Follow the instructions on your kit, and add your preferred synergy of essential oils to the melted wax before you place the wax into the mould.

✳ A good blend for enticing the appetite is bay (which has a sweet and spicy, cinnamon-like aroma), bitter orange and sweet thyme.

✳ If the atmosphere has become too stimulating, and your guests show no signs of departing, extinguish the flame of a nearby candle, add 3 drops of lavender to the melted wax and re-light. The lavender blends excellently with the synergy mix, and is soothing enough for your guests to start feeling a little sleepy and ready to go home.

Caution: Essential oils are highly flammable, so never add them to a lighted candle flame, because it will flare up and can cause a serious burn. Keep the wick trimmed short; if the flame is too high, it will not reach the melted pool of wax below to lift the vapour of the essential oil. The pool of wax needs to be big and the wick short to diffuse the essential oil.

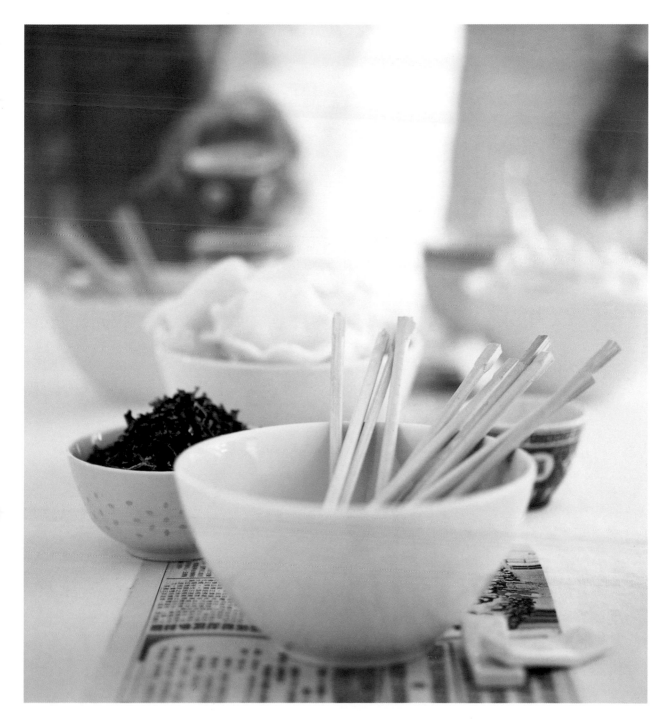

Lounge

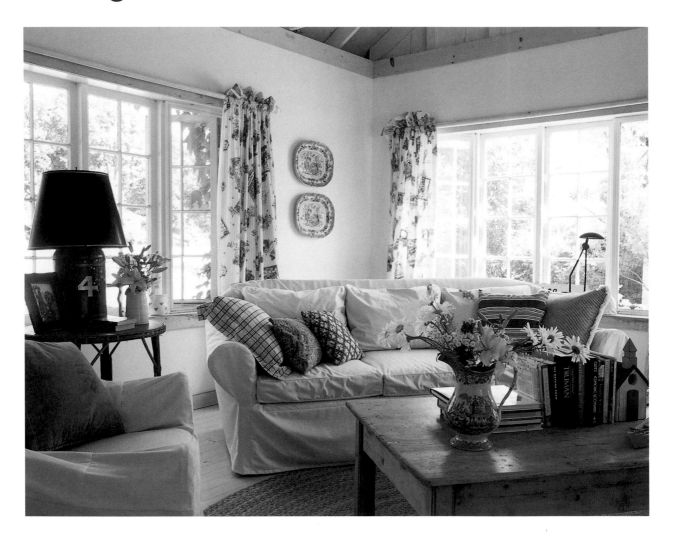

Using the natural smells of essential oils, rather than the commercially available synthetic perfumes or air fresheners, in your living area will provide you with harmonious aromas that will relax and stimulate you in equal measure.

Using essential oils in a plant mist-sprayer (see page 105) is an effective way to freshen up furniture, curtains and carpets, but remember to avoid spraying wood, velvet and silk, because water stains may occur due to the strength of the oils.

Recommended essential oils

Bergamot, cedarwood (Atlas and Virginian), clary sage, cypress, elemi, lavender, lemon grass, patchouli, pine, rose and sandalwood.

Methods of use

Carpet freshener

This blend is very refreshing, kills airborne germs and acts as an insect-repellent.

＊ 225g (8oz) bicarbonate of soda
＊ 20 drops elemi
＊ 10 drops lemon grass
＊ 10 drops patchouli

Place the bicarbonate of soda with the synergistic blend of essential oils in a sealed container and keep for at least 24 hours. Sprinkle over the carpet and leave for half an hour before vacuum-cleaning the carpet. Do not empty the dust from the vacuum-cleaner until absolutely necessary, because the aroma will penetrate the vacuum-cleaner and continue to provide fragrance every time you clean.

Furniture polish

＊ 25g (1oz) yellow unrefined beeswax
＊ 125ml (4fl oz) turpentine
＊ 13 drops lavender
＊ 2 drops patchouli

Grate the beeswax, and heat it in a basin over a pan of warm water until completely melted. Remove from the heat and immediately stir in the turpentine, before the wax begins to set, making sure that it is thoroughly mixed. Then stir in the essential oils.

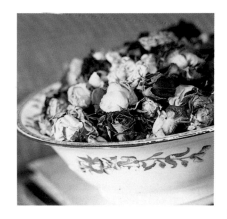

When cooled, keep the mixture in a sealed glass pot. Use only a very tiny amount on your cloth and buff with a clean duster.

Caution: Never add turpentine to the basin while the pan is still on the heat, as it is highly flammable.

Room fresheners

For a warm, soothing atmosphere, use the following blend:

＊ 300ml (10fl oz) rose floral water
＊ 3 drops bergamot
＊ 5 drops clary sage
＊ 2 drops sandalwood

For a fresh, clean, uplifting atmosphere, use the following blend:

＊ 300ml (10fl oz) peppermint floral water
＊ 3 drops cedarwood
＊ 5 drops cypress
＊ 2 drops pine

Pot pourri

You can make your own pot pourri by collecting all types of dried herbs, wood shavings, dried fruit and their stones, leaves, nutmegs, nuts, pine cones, cinnamon sticks, cloves and flower petals.

Citrus fruit peel also makes a great addition to pot pourri. To dry the peel, you should wrap it in a kitchen towel and place it in a microwave oven for a few seconds. This will dry and curl the peel into beautiful shapes, ready for use in your pot pourri.

How to make pot pourri

＊ Mix 1 tablespoon of orrisroot powder with 10 drops of your choice of essential oils.

＊ Put around 300g (10oz) of the mixed pot pourri in a plastic bag with the orrisroot and the essential oils.

＊ Keep the mixture in a sealed bag for two days, allowing the essential oils to penetrate the pot pourri. Then put the mixture into an attractive bowl.

Bathroom

The bathroom needs to be clean and free from bacteria, especially if the toilet is in the bathroom. The synergistic blend below is an excellent disinfectant and anti-bacterial agent, and will also help keep mould out of the bathroom. When you are happy that your bathroom is clean and fresh, there is nothing better than taking a leisurely bath enhanced with essential oils, whether the purpose of this is simple relaxation or to stimulate the senses.

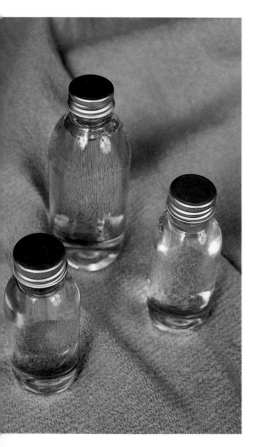

Recommended essential oils

Bergamot, Roman camomile, elemi, jasmine, lavender, lemon, lime, niaouli, sweet orange, tea tree, sweet thyme and ylang ylang.

Methods of use

Bathroom cleaner

✳ 300ml (10fl oz) water
✳ 10 drops elemi
✳ 10 drops lemon
✳ 10 drops lime
✳ 10 drops niaouli
✳ 10 drops tea tree
✳ 10 drops sweet thyme

Blend all the ingredients and pour into a spray bottle. Shake the bottle and spray around and inside the toilet, the sink, the bath, the shower and around the shower curtain. Leave for a few minutes and then rinse off. This blend is also excellent for getting rid of mould on tiles and shower curtains.

Diffusing oils

For safety reasons, never use an electric diffuser in the bathroom. Use a conventional oil burner or try dropping essential oils straight onto the cardboard ring of the toilet paper. Bergamot, pine, lemon and lime make a good blend for this purpose.

Foam and milk bath bases

To make up a bath blend, you will need unscented foam and milk bath bases which are available from any good supplier of aromatherapy products.

Milk bath bases are non-foaming dispersing agents suitable for use with essential oils. As they are more gentle than foam bases, it is advisable to use them when adding essential oils to the bath for very young children and babies.

Bath blends

When making up the blends suggested below, use bottles that match or complement the colour of your bathroom, because they make lovely decorations when not in use.

✳ Relaxing preparation: 500ml (17fl oz) foam or milk bath base, 12 drops bergamot, 16 drops Roman camomile, 2 drops jasmine.

✳ Sensual preparation: 500ml (17fl oz) foam or milk bath base, 15 drops lavender, 10 drops sweet orange, 5 drops ylang ylang.

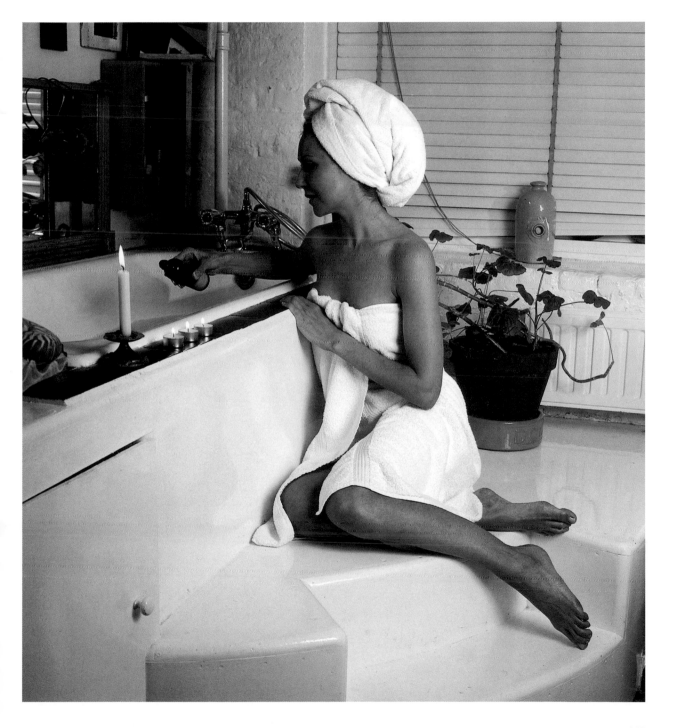

Bedroom

This room is normally associated with peace, rest, tranquillity and romance. It can be full of soft and vibrant colours, flowers and fragrant cushions. The essential oils that spring to mind for creating a calming ambience in the bedroom are clary sage, jasmine, rose and ylang ylang. This combination can be used in a room spray and regularly sprayed in the room.

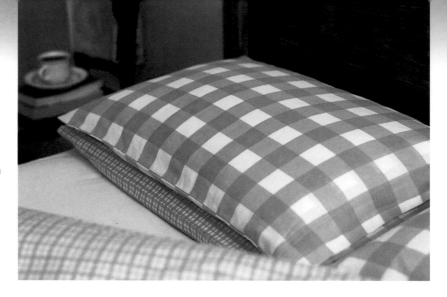

Recommended essential oils

Bergamot, Roman camomile, clary sage, jasmine, lavender, neroli and sandalwood.

Methods of use

Fragrant cushions

Cushions for placing on the bed can be filled with dried herbs and perfumed with any essential oils that you enjoy. Just stitch three sides of any size of fabric, and stuff with herbs that have been treated with essential oils. Stitch the final side together, and put this inner cushion into a plain cover filled with soft packing material to make it more comfortable. Now, cover the completed herb cushion with a pretty cover, and place it on the bed. Every time you lean on the cushion, the smell will burst forth. When the smell starts to disappear, just replenish the herbs with more essential oils.

Infusing bed linen

The bed linen can also be infused with essential oils while it is in the airing cupboard. Drop as many drops of your favourite essential oils as you need on strips of fabric and place these in between your bed linen. The aroma from the strips of fabric will infuse into the bed linen.

Synergistic blends for the bedroom

These can be used in room sprays (see page 105), in fragrant cushions or for infusing bed linen.

✳ Deep sleep: 3 drops Roman camomile, 3 drops lavender, 2 drops neroli, 1 drop sandalwood.

✳ Romance: 3 drops bergamot, 6 drops clary sage, 1 drop jasmine.

Keeping clothes and shoes fresh

When storing clothes, a good synergistic blend for keeping them fresh and repelling moths is 2 drops of citronella , 3 drops of lavender and 2 drops of lemon grass. Place this mixture on the inside or middle of cottonwool balls and hook these onto the clothes-hangers, or in between the clothes if they are stored in drawers. Alternatively, put the drops of essential oils on some absorbent kitchen paper and place the sheet on the bottom of the drawer.

For smelly shoes, add 5 drops of lemon grass to cottonwool balls and leave the cotton balls in the shoes overnight. The shoes will smell fresh and clean the next day.

Child's bedroom

This is their room and it should show their own individual personality; you cannot compel your children to have your taste in decoration. Encourage them to design and take an interest in what is their own domain. This will help them to take pride in their room and keep it clean and tidy. Smell is an important factor in our lives. We want our children to feel secure and happy, so introducing aromas into their room will have a cheering effect on their emotions, which will last into their adulthood. Lemon, lime, mandarin

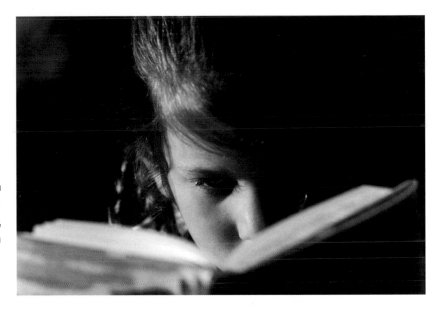

Papier-mâché mobile

Add a few drops of your child's favourite aroma to a paste made from flour and water. Using layers of paper and paste, fashion some interesting shapes. Pierce a hole through each shape with a warm needle, allow the shapes to dry and then paint them. Add essential oils to the paint for a penetrating aroma. Attach the shapes with thread or string to a framework made from metal or cardboard. When the mobile is hung up, the natural heat generated from the room, will release the aroma.

and sweet orange are aromas that children usually like.

Start when the child is young by decorating the room with papier-mâché mobiles (see panel). Favourite cushions, soft toys and paper objects can all be infused with aroma by placing them in a polythene bag together with cottonwool balls filled with essential oils. Leave for a day or two, and then place the infused items around the child's room.

The bedroom as a study

There will come a time when teenagers will need to use their bedroom as a study. This can be an emotional and stressful time for them. Encourage them to vaporize essential oils in their room for the study periods only. This will allow the

temporal neocortex (the part of the brain responsible for long-term memory) to associate the aroma with the study. An excellent blend for study is basil and rosemary: just put 3 drops of each onto a diffuser and vaporize the room. If they have a particularly difficult subject to revise for, this blend will aid memory. When they are ready to sit their exam, put 1 drop of each on a handkerchief for them to smell during the exam; this will help them to concentrate on the study they did previously.

Relaxing may also be a problem during this time. When your child is ready to relax, change the aroma to a more calming one. Blend 2 drops of bergamot, 1 drop of frankincense and 3 drops of petitgrain. This will help calm anxiety, and aid sleep.

Directory of essential oils

Name	Note	Part(s) of plant used	Properties and uses	Special points
Angelica (*Angelica archangelica*)	Base note	Seed, root	Good for fatigue, migraine, nervous tension, stress-related disorders, muscular aches and pains, accumulation of toxins and dull, congested skin.	*Caution:* Highly phototoxic; keep out of the sun.
Basil (*Ocimum basilicum* ct. linalol)	Top note	Flowering top, leaf	Treats insect bites (mosquito, wasp), gout, muscular aches and pains, rheumatism, bronchitis, coughs, earache, sinusitis, dyspepsia, flatulence, nausea, cramps, irregular periods, colds, fever, flu and infectious diseases.	*Caution:* Maximum use level is 2 per cent.
Bay (*Pimenta racemosa*)	Top note	Dried leaf	Good for muscular aches and pains, neuralgia, rheumatism and poor circulation. Excellent for the scalp and all hair conditions. Builds up the immune system.	*Caution:* Do not use if taking aspirin, heparin or warfarin.
Benzoin (*Styrax benzoin*)	Base note	Gum	Very warming. Excellent for dry and cracked skin. Tonic for the lungs, and beneficial for respiratory disorders, bronchitis, asthma, coughs, colds and laryngitis. Soothing and uplifting, it is helpful for people suffering from low spirits or mild depression.	
Bergamot (*Citrus bergamia*)	Top note	Fruit peel	Sedative, yet uplifting. Used mainly for infections, depression and anxiety. Excellent for skin care, helping with psoriasis, acne, eczema and varicose ulcers. Helpful as a preventative for cystitis and ongoing illnesses.	*Caution:* Photosensitive; keep out of the sun.
Cajuput (*Melaleuca leucadendron*)	Top note	Leaf, twig	Treats rheumatism, arthritis, muscular aches and pains, gout, varicose veins, insect bites and oily skin. Clearing for asthma, catarrh, constipation and flatulence. Builds up the immune system.	*Caution:* Care is advisable in pregnancy.
Camomile, German (*Matricaria chamomilla*)	Middle note	Dried flower	Good for all skin conditions, such as skin allergies, wounds, ulcers, eczema, sensitive skin and fungal infections. Useful for inflamed and swollen joints.	
Camomile, Roman (*Chamaemelum nobile*)	Middle note	Flower	Sedative, soothing. Beneficial for menstrual pain, arthritis, nerve pain, headaches, eczema, dermatitis, acne and allergic conditions. Good for dry and itchy skin. Excellent skin cleanser. Safe for children.	*Caution:* Avoid in early pregnancy.
Cardamom (*Elettaria cardamomum*)	Top to middle note	Dried ripe fruit	Warming to the mind, and eases stomach cramp, colic, flatulence and heartburn.	
Carrot seed (*Daucus carota*)	Top to middle note	Seed	Good for skin conditions such as dermatitis, eczema and psoriasis, and nourishing to mature skin.	
Cedarwood, Atlas (*Cedrus atlantica*)	Base note	Wood	Tonic action on the glandular and nervous systems helps put the body back into balance. Antiseptic and diuretic, which can help with cellulite. Treats bronchitis and catarrh, relieving aching muscles. Toning effect on the skin, useful for acne.	

Name	Note	Part(s) of plant used	Properties and uses	Special points
Cedarwood, Virginian (*Juniperus virginiana*)	Base note	Wood	Excellent antiseptic properties. Beneficial for acne, dandruff, eczema, ulcers and oily skin.	
Celery seed (*Apium graveolens*)	Top to middle note	Fruit, seed	Sedative and tonic effect on the central nervous system. Clears toxins within the body. Tonic for the digestive system and reproductive system.	**Caution:** *Avoid during pregnancy.*
Cinnamon leaf (*Cinnamomum zeylanicum*)	Base note	Leaf	Good for the digestive system. Calms spasms, colitis, flatulence, diarrhoea and nausea. Stimulates secretions of gastric juices. Eases muscular spasms and painful rheumatic joints, aches and pains.	**Caution:** *Avoid in pregnancy. It is a powerful oil so use with care.*
Citronella (*Cymbopogon nardus*)	Top note	Leaf	Excellent insect-repellent. Its deodorizing and stimulating properties refresh sweaty, tired feet.	**Caution:** *Can cause skin sensitization.*
Clary sage (*Salvia sclarea*)	Top note	Flower	Euphoric. Good for depression, panicky states, menstrual disorders, cramp, pre-menstrual syndrome, high blood pressure and period pain. Excellent for relaxing muscles. Soothing action relieves headaches and migraine by calming tension. Not to be confused with common sage (*Salvia officinalis*) which is not to be used in aromatherapy.	**Caution:** *Avoid in early pregnancy.*
Clove (*Syzygium aromaticum*)	Base note	Bud	Painkiller. Good for rheumatoid arthritis, toothache, neuralgia, gum infections, infected acne, ulcers and wounds. Antiseptic. Good for prevention of disease, cystitis, diarrhoea and sinusitis. Can be helpful for Crohn's disease and low immunity. It has hormonal qualities, so is useful for thyroid imbalance.	**Caution:** *Irritant to the skin in high dosage levels.*
Coriander (*Coriandrum sativum*)	Top note	Fruit, seed	Helps with migraine, neuralgia, nervous exhaustion, muscular aches and pains, accumulation of toxins and poor circulation. Tonic for the immune system.	
Cypress (*Cupressus sempervirens*)	Middle note	Leaf, cone	Antiseptic and diuretic. Good for circulation, cellulite and varicose veins. Will improve skin tone and help eliminate toxins. Slightly astringent, so good for oily skin.	
Elemi (*Canarium luzonicum*)	Middle to base note	Bark	Good for colds and flu. With its antiseptic properties, it is also good for infected cuts and wounds.	
Eucalyptus (*Eucalyptus citriodora*)	Top note	Leaf	Insect-repellent. Good for skin fungal infections, such as athlete's foot, and dandruff.	**Caution:** *May cause skin sensitization.*
Eucalyptus (*Eucalyptus globulus*)	Top note	Leaf	Stimulant, antiseptic and anti-inflammatory. Treats respiratory tract, and is useful for sinusitis and head colds. Eases rheumatism, arthritis and muscular aches and pains.	**Caution:** *Contraindicated for very young children and babies because of its high cineole content.*

Name	Note	Part(s) of plant used	Properties and uses	Special points
Eucalyptus (*Eucalyptus smithii*)	Top note	Leaf	Good for headaches and migraines, warming to muscle aches and pains and beneficial for colds, catarrh, coughs, sinusitis and asthma.	
Fennel (*Foeniculum vulgare*)	Middle note	Seed	Excellent body cleanser, ridding the system of toxins. Good for hangovers. Diuretic, helpful in reducing diets and for cellulite. Tonic for the digestion, easing indigestion, constipation and flatulence. Good for pre-menstrual syndrome, irregular periods, menopausal problems and low sexual response. Helps cleanse and tone the skin.	***Caution:*** *Not recommended for young children. Avoid in pregnancy. Do not use if epileptic. Best avoided in alcoholism and liver disease, and if taking paracetamol owing to anethole (toxic) content.*
Frankincense (*Boswellia carteri*)	Base note	Bark	Balancing. Helps with stress and nervous tension. Used in facial oils to deter fine lines and wrinkles. Helps with rheumatoid arthritis, and good for asthma.	
Galbanum (*Ferula galbaniflua*)	Top note	Bark	Relieves stress. Good for aches and pains, and for poor circulation. Toning to the skin, and cleansing for acne, boils and scar tissue.	
Geranium (*Pelargonium graveolens*)	Middle note	Flower, leaf	Balancing. Helps with period pains, menopausal problems, mood swings, cold sores, shingles, skin problems and anxiety. Revitalizes the body and regulates hormonal balance.	***Caution:*** *May cause skin sensitization in hypersensitive individuals.*
Ginger (*Zingiber officinale*)	Top note	Rhizome	Good for catarrh, congestion, coughs, sore throat, diarrhoea, colic, cramp, flatulence, indigestion and loss of appetite. Warming for muscular aches and pains, arthritis and poor circulation. Can help with chills, colds and flu. Relieves nervous exhaustion.	
Grapefruit (*Citrus paradisi*)	Top note	Fruit peel	Euphoric, refreshing, anti-depressant, immune stimulant and lymphatic stimulant. Good for cellulite.	***Caution:*** *Photosensitive; keep out of the sun.*
Ho leaf (*Cinnamomum camphora* ct. *linalol*)	Base note	Wood, leaf	Helps with acne, dermatitis, scars, wounds, wrinkles and general skin care. Not to be confused with ho wood, which is not to be used in aromatherapy.	
Immortelle (*Helichrysum angustifolia*)	Middle to base note	Flower	Good for depression, shock, fears and phobias, as well as general aches and pains. Its cell-regenerating properties make it useful for scars, acne, dermatitis and abscesses. Good for colds and flu.	

Name	Note	Part(s) of plant used	Properties and uses	Special points
Jasmine absolute (*Jasminum grandiflorum*)	Base note	Flower	Emotionally warming and uplifting, euphoric. Eases depression, postnatal depression, lack of confidence and emotional imbalance. Soothes and hydrates dry skin.	**Caution:** *Not to be used in pregnancy.*
Juniper berry (*Juniperus communis*)	Middle note	Berry	Clears, stimulates and strengthens the nerves. Very strong diuretic and antiseptic, valuable in cystitis, cellulite and fluid retention. Detoxifies and cleanses the body. Eliminates uric acid and helps in cases of arthritis, rheumatism and gout. A tonic for oily and congested skins, easing acne, blocked pores, dermatitis, weeping eczema, psoriasis and swellings.	**Caution:** *Over-stimulating for the kidneys, and best avoided during early pregnancy.*
Lavandin (*Lavandula x intermedia*)	Top note	Flower	Good for circulation, respiratory and muscle problems.	**Caution:** *Use with care because of its camphor content, which is higher than that of true lavender oil. Avoid in pregnancy, and with epilepsy or fever.*
Lavender (*Lavandula angustifolia*)	Middle note	Flower	True lavender is the most versatile of all the oils. There are many variations within the species depending on where it is grown (see page 10). Sedative, antiseptic, antibiotic, anti-viral and anti-fungal. Treats burns, abrasions, coughs, colds, flu, stress, nausea, ulcers, acne, asthma, insect bites, rheumatism, arthritis, headaches, migraine and insomnia.	**Caution:** *Avoid in early pregnancy.*
Lavender, spike (*Lavandula latifolia*)	Top note	Flower	Helps clear a stuffy head and makes the senses calmer, yet more alert. Particularly effective for bronchitis and headaches linked to catarrh. Helps build up the immune system to protect against viral attacks. Excellent for muscular aches and pains. Cleansing for the skin, and has fungicidal properties.	**Caution:** *Use with care because of its camphor content, which is higher than that of true lavender oil. Avoid in pregnancy, and with epilepsy or fever.*
Lemon (*Citrus limon*)	Top note	Fruit peel	Eases anxiety, depression and confusion. Brings cheer and strength in times of illness and convalescence. Stimulant for the immune and nervous system. Assists purification of the blood and lymphatic system. Tonic for the liver, gallbladder, pancreas and circulatory system. Antiseptic properties, aiding healing of wounds and infections. Digestive aid. Counteracts acidity and cholesterol build-up in the body.	**Caution:** *Photosensitive; keep out of the sun.*

Name	Note	Part(s) of plant used	Properties and uses	Special points
Lemon grass (*Cymbopogon citratus*)	Top note	Leaf	Excellent insect-repellent. With its deodorizing and antiseptic properties, it is good for athlete's foot and excessive perspiration.	
Lime (*Citrus aurantifolia*)	Top note	Fruit peel	Relieves anxiety and depression. Good for use when convalescing after an illness.	*Caution:* Photosensitive; keep out of the sun.
Mandarin (*Citrus reticulata*)	Top note	Fruit peel	Good for nervous tension, fluid retention and oily or congested skin. Helpful for stretch marks.	
Manuka (*Leptospermum scoparium*)	Top note	Leaf, branchlet	Warming, invigorating for the mind and body. Used for meditation. Beneficial for rheumatoid arthritis, acne, dermatitis and allergenic rashes, bronchitis, sinusitis and asthma.	*Caution:* Moderate skin irritant; may cause redness and soreness when applied undiluted.
Marjoram, Spanish (*Thymus mastichina*)	Middle note	Leaf	Good for sinusitis, catarrh and viral and bacterial infections. Warming and cleansing for muscles.	
Marjoram, sweet (*Origanum majorana*)	Middle note	Flowerhead, leaf	Sedative, good for asthma, constipation and high blood pressure. Anaphrodisiac. Good for muscular spasms, migraine, aches and pains.	*Caution:* Avoid in early pregnancy.
May chang (*Litsea cubeba*)	Top note	Fruit	Uplifting and stimulating. Tonic for the heart and respiratory system. Beneficial effect on coronary heart disease. Balancing action on oily skin and hair.	*Caution:* Do not use on diseased, damaged or hypersensitive, skin, or for children under 2 years old.
Melissa, true (*Melissa officinalis*)	Middle note	Flower, leaf	Good for insomnia, and calming to the nervous system. Useful for digestive problems such as stomach cramp, nausea and morning sickness.	
Myrrh (*Commiphora myrrha*)	Base note	Stem, branch	Antiseptic and fungicidal properties. Assists the healing of wounds, and is good for the throat, mouth and gums. Stimulates digestion. Aids respiratory problems such as bronchitis, colds, catarrh and sore throat. Rejuvenates aged skin.	*Caution:* Not to be used in early pregnancy.
Myrtle (*Myrtus communis*)	Middle note	Leaf, twig	Beneficial for asthma, bronchitis, catarrhal conditions, chronic coughs, colds, flu and infectious diseases.	
Neroli (*Citrus aurantium* var. *amara*)	Base note	Flower	Boosts confidence and self-esteem. Relaxing, powerful aid for relieving mental or emotional stress and anxiety. Eases fear, depression, grief, shock and hysteria. Gentle and relaxing aphrodisiac. Treats insomnia, promoting deep and restful sleep. Rejuvenating and soothing for skin care.	

Name	Note	Part(s) of plant used	Properties and uses	Special points
Niaouli (*Melaleuca viridiflora*)	Top note	Leaf, shoot	Tissue stimulant, promoting local circulation, increasing white blood cell and antibody activity, helping to fight infections. Helps weakened conditions. Good to use at the beginning of an illness since it helps to strengthen the immune system. Good for chest infections, bronchitis, flu, pneumonia, whooping cough, asthma, sinusitis, catarrh, laryngitis, urinary infections. For skin care, it can firm the tissues and aids healing.	*Caution:* Use with care in pregnancy, and for young children.
Orange, bitter (*Citrus aurantium* var. *amara*)	Top note	Fruit peel	Promotes mental clarity and emotional balance. Good for constipation, aiding muscular spasms, lymphatic drainage and fluid retention.	*Caution:* Photosensitive; keep out of the sun.
Orange, sweet (*Citrus aurantium* var. *sinensis*)	Top note	Fruit peel	Sedative, warming properties make it helpful for depression or nervous tension. Good for colds, flu, fluid retention and obesity. Eases bronchitis, and has a calming effect on the stomach, aiding constipation and indigestion.	
Palmarosa (*Cymbopogon martinii*)	Top note	Leaf	Clears the mind. Antiseptic, hydrating and soothing for the skin. Vitalizes and regenerates skin cells. Beneficial for acne and other skin problems. Stimulates digestion. Anti-viral properties.	
Patchouli (*Pogostemon patchouli*)	Base note	Leaf	Aphrodisiac, easing impotence and frigidity. Alleviates lethargy, confusion and depression, and calms stress and anxiety. Sedative, antiseptic, anti-fungal and anti-bacterial properties. Regenerates skin cells, so is useful for aged skin, cracked skin, acne, dandruff, eczema and other skin problems.	
Pepper, black (*Piper nigrum*)	Middle note	Berry	Stimulates, strengthens the nerves and mind and gives stamina. Tonic for skeletal muscles. Good for muscular aches and pains, and for use before excessive sport. Stimulates appetite, expels wind and can be stimulating for the circulation. Has a beneficial effect on respiratory illnesses.	
Peppermint (*Mentha x piperita*)	Top note	Leaf, flowering top	Refreshing, stimulates the mind and aids concentration. Excellent for motion sickness, headaches and nausea. Highly beneficial for digestive disorders. Good for fever, colds and flu. Antiseptic, cleansing for the skin. Helps relieve muscle, arthritic and menstrual pain.	*Caution:* Contraindicated for babies and young children, where it can produce laryngospasm (closure of the larynx). Can cause skin irritation. Do not use if taking homeopathic remedies.

Name	Note	Part(s) of plant used	Properties and uses	Special points
Petitgrain (*Citrus aurantium* var. *amara*)	Middle note	Leaf	Clears the mind and eases mental fatigue. Aids insomnia and stimulates the digestive processes. Sedative of the nervous system. Tonic effect on the skin, which could help clear up skin blemishes such as pimples or acne.	
Pine (*Pinus sylvestris*)	Top note	Needle	Uplifting for nervous exhaustion and fatigue. Helps with poor circulation, bronchitis, catarrh, asthma and sinusitis. Excellent for vaporizing when there is illness, because it can kill airborne germs.	
Ravensara (*Ravensara aromatica*)	Middle note	Leaf	Tonic for the immune system, and helpful with glandular fever. Anti-fungal, antiseptic. Helpful with chicken pox, herpes, muscle aches and pains. Good for bronchitis, flu, sinusitis and whooping cough.	
Rose otto (*Rosa damascena*)	Base note	Flower	Gentle aphrodisiac, aiding impotence and frigidity. Relieves tension, depression, postnatal depression, sadness and grief. Regulates the female reproductive system, and is especially beneficial for the uterus. Powerful tonic effect upon the circulation, nervous system and digestion. Aids regeneration of skin cells, so is excellent for skin problems and general skin care.	
Rosemary (*Rosmarinus officinalis*)	Middle note	Flowerhead, leaf	Stimulant. Good for muscular aches and pains, poor circulation, rheumatic problems, physical and mental fatigue, low blood pressure and hair loss.	***Caution:*** *Do not use if epileptic, with high blood pressure or in the early stages of pregnancy. Not normally used on those inclined to liver problems.*
Sandalwood (*Santalum album*)	Base note	Heartwood	Promotes deep, peaceful meditation. Relaxing and calming, easing depression, stress and fear. Aphrodisiac. Stimulates and strengthens the immune system, and is beneficial for urinary infections. Soothes sore throats, and helps ease laryngitis and bronchitis. Soothing and moisturizing for dry skin; antiseptic and astringent for oily skin and acne.	
Tagétes (*Tagetes glandulifera*)	Middle note	Flower	Anti-fungal, therefore good for candida infection. Good for catarrhal infections, wound healing, bronchitis and coughs.	***Caution:*** *Do not use on children or babies, and avoid in pregnancy. Phototoxic; keep out of the sun.*

Name	Note	Part(s) of plant used	Properties and uses	Special points
Tea tree (*Melaleuca alternifolia*)	Top note	Leaf	Stimulant. Good for candida infection, thrush, nail bed infections, athlete's foot, cold sores, mouth ulcers, immune system, acne, spots, bites and stings. Beneficial for the respiratory system, easing colds, flu, asthma and bronchitis. Its fungicidal properties help clear thrush and are of value with genital infections generally. Also a urinary tract antiseptic, alleviating problems such as cystitis.	*Caution:* May cause irritation on sensitive areas of skin if over-used.
Thyme, red (*Thymus vulgaris* ct. thymol)	Top note	Flower, leaf	Anti-bacterial, anti-fungal. Good for acne, boils, skin problems, circulatory disorders, hair loss, flatulence, sluggish digestion, bronchial secretions, sinusitis, asthma, general fatigue, hypertension, depression, examination nerves, anxiety and, because of its warming properties, rheumatism and stiff joints.	*Caution:* Do not use with high blood pressure. Irritant to the skin.
Thyme, sweet (*Thymus vulgaris* ct. geraniol, ct. linalol)	Top note	Flower, leaf	Good for bronchitis, sinusitis, cystitis, muscular rheumatism, dry eczema, psoriasis, weeping eczema, sore throat, tonsillitis, colitis and infected acne. Can help people who are prone to viral attacks, fatigue and insomnia.	
Valerian (*Valeriana officinalis*)	Base note	Rhizome, root	Helps with insomnia, migraine, restlessness and nervous tension. Eases high blood pressure and nervous indigestion.	
Vetiver (*Vetiveria zizanioides*)	Base note	Root	Good for general infections, skin infections, acne, infrequent (or loss of) periods and diabetes.	
Yarrow (*Achillea millefolium*)	Base note	Dried flowerhead	Good all-round oil that benefits insomnia, stress-related conditions, high blood pressure, acne, eczema, wounds, colds, fever and flu.	*Caution:* Avoid in early pregnancy.
Ylang ylang (*Cananga odorata*)	Base note	Flower	Relaxing aphrodisiac, euphoric. Good for high blood pressure, impotence, frigidity, pre-menstrual syndrome, depression, irritability, panic attacks and hypersensitive states. Stimulates hair growth. Balances oily skin.	*Caution:* Slight risk of skin sensitization.

Directory of carrier oils

Name	Note	Properties and uses	Special points
Almond, sweet (*Prunus amygdalis* var. *dulcis*)	Cold-pressed	The sweet almond tree yields a fixed oil obtained by cold-pressing. It contains vitamins A, B1, B2, B6 and E. Because of its small amount of vitamin E, it keeps reasonably well. It protects and nourishes the skin, and calms the irritation caused by eczema, psoriasis, dermatitis and all cases of dry scaly skin. It has been known to help with irritation on babies' bottoms, and soothes sunburn.	***Caution:*** *Can be contraindicated for nut allergy.*
Apricot kernel (*Prunus armeniaca*)	Cold-pressed	Apricot oil is almost identical to sweet almond. Less oil is produced, however, making it slightly more expensive. Apricot is excellent for skin protection, being both emollient and nourishing. It is readily absorbed into the skin because of its light texture. It calms irritation caused by eczema, and is suitable for sensitive, dry and ageing skins.	
Avocado (*Persea americana*)	Cold-pressed	The unrefined oil should be rich green in colour and is pressed from the dried and sliced flesh from fruits. Contains vitamins A, B1, B2 and D. It is a superb emollient, and has a reputation for having a higher degree of penetration into the epidermis than most carrier oils. Avocado has excellent skin-healing properties, and it is beneficial for very dry skin and wrinkles.	
Borage (*Borago officinalis*)	Cold-pressed	With levels of 16–23 per cent, borage is the richest source of GLA (gamma-linolenic acid) currently available. It is non-irritant, so may be used on the skin in cases of eczema and psoriasis, and helps soften wrinkles. GLA is a natural substance made by the body's own healthy cells, and is found in hemp, borage and evening primrose oils. It helps conditions such as arthritis and pre-menstrual syndrome, where the body's ability to make GLA acid is impaired.	
Calendula (*Calendula officinalis*)	Macerated in sunflower oil	This excellent healing oil is good for bed sores, broken veins, bruises, stubborn wounds and varicose veins. It is excellent for skin problems, particularly rashes, chapped and cracked skin and dry eczema.	
Camellia (*Camellia sinensis*)	Macerated in sunflower oil	Camellia is the tea plant grown in eastern Asia. It is used in traditional Chinese medicine for treating skin conditions. It is very good for very sensitive and mature skin.	
Carrot (*Daucus carota*)	Macerated in sunflower oil	True carrot oil is rich in beta-carotene and vitamins A, B, C, D, E and F. It is an excellent tonic for the skin, helping the healing process by assisting in the formation of scar tissue. It soothes itching skin and is helpful in cases of psoriasis and eczema. It is particularly good for delaying the ageing process.	
Coconut (*Cocos nucifera*)	Cold-pressed	The oil is frequently used in massage creams because of its skin-softening properties. Coconut oil makes the skin smooth and satin-like. It is excellent for conditioning the hair.	
Evening primrose (*Oenothera biennis*)	Cold-pressed	Rich in GLA (see Borage, above), this oil is helpful for psoriasis, dry scaly skin and dandruff, and accelerates wound healing.	
Grapeseed (*Vitis vinifera*)	Refined	A light, non-greasy massage oil.	

Name	Note	Properties and uses	Special points
Hypericum or St John's wort (*Hypericum perforatum*)	Macerated in sunflower oil	Hypericum is particularly soothing to inflamed nerves, making it helpful for cases of neuralgia, sciatica and fibrositis. It is good for wounds where there is nerve-tissue damage, and is effective for sprains, burns and bruises. It is excellent for the skin, since it is soothing and antiseptic. It is used in cosmetics to tighten the skin.	
Jojoba (*Simmondsia chinensis*)	Cold-pressed	Jojoba is not an oil but a liquid wax. The chemical structure of jojoba not only resembles sebum (see page 17), but the latter can dissolve in it, which makes it useful in cases of acne. Good for dry scalp and skin, psoriasis and eczema, it is a very balancing oil.	
Macadamia (*Macadamia ternifolia*)	Cold-pressed	Macadamia has good keeping properties. It is a skin lubricant and is easily absorbed by the skin. Macadamia has very similar properties to human skin, making it beneficial for rejuvenating ageing skin. It is also non-greasy and has been described as a 'vanishing' oil.	
Neem seed (*Melia azadiracta*)	Cold-pressed	The neem tree is part of a genus of big tropical trees that yield valuable timber. The fruit is a capsule, with a few large seeds with fleshy jackets. Neem is effective in the treatment of skin diseases such as psoriasis, eczema, dermatitis, burns, ulcers, herpes and fungal infections, as well as warts and dandruff. It has anti-inflammatory properties, making it beneficial for arthritis and aches and pains, and is reported to be anti-bacterial. It is used extensively in India as an insect-repellent and organic insecticide.	
Peach kernel (*Amygdalus persica*)	Cold-pressed	Physically, peach kernel oil is similar to apricot kernel and sweet almond oils. It has good skin-protection qualities, is emollient and nourishing and is slowly absorbed. It relieves itching and is beneficial for eczema. Peach kernel is suitable for sensitive, dry and ageing skins and makes a good facial massage oil. It is often used in skin-care creams.	
Rose hip (*Rosa canina*)	Cold-pressed	This may be used in cosmetic creams and lotions. It has been found that the oil is a tissue-regenerator, helping to prevent premature ageing, minimize wrinkles and reduce scar tissue. It is also useful for burns and eczema.	
Sunflower (*Helianthus annuus*)	Cold-pressed	This is produced from oil obtained by organically grown plants. It contains vitamins A, B, D and E. It has a soothing effect on the skin and is beneficial for leg ulcers, bruises and skin diseases.	***Caution:*** *Do not use supermarket sunflower oil, as this is refined oil for cooking only, which has had any moisturizing and healing properties removed.*
Wheatgerm (*Triticum vulgare*)	Cold-pressed	Rich orange in colour due to its high vitamin E content, this oil is useful for dry and mature skins, and is excellent for stretch marks and scar tissue.	***Caution:*** *Contrainidicated for allergies.*

Index

Acknowledgements

Bridgeman Art Library, London/New York /British Museum, London, UK 12, /The Stapleton Collection 8.

Garden Picture Library /Ron Evans 58, /Jerry Pavia 89

Gattefossé s.a 13.

Getty Images /Britt Erlanson 92.

Octopus Publishing Group Limited /Colin Bowling 20, 25, 55, 57, 62, 66, 71, 73, 77, 78, 93, 95, 97, 98, 99, 100, /Jerry Harpur 11, /Rupert Horrox 114, /Sandra Lane 67, 86, /Gary Latham 56, /Di Lewis 104, /William Lingwood 105, /David Loftus 103, /Peter Myers 26–27, 28, 34 top, 35, 35 bottom, 36 top, 36 bottom, 37 top right, 60, /Peter Pugh-Cook 14, 23, 74, 81, 112, 113, /William Reavell 15, 19, 82, 91, 101, 109, /Paul Ryan 110, /Gareth Sambidge 21, 24, 29, 30 top centre, 30 top left, 30 top right, 30 bottom centre, 32, 33, 34 bottom centre, 38 left, 38 right, 39 top left, 39 top right, 39 bottom right, 40, 41 left, 41 right, 42, 43 left, 43 right, 43 centre, 45 top left, 45 top right, 45 bottom right, 45 bottom left, 48, 49 top right, 49 bottom left, 50, 51, 52, 59, 64, 70, 79, 85, 88, /Roger Stowell 69, 96, /Richard Truscott 87, /Ian Wallace back cover, 6, 9, 10, 22, 37 top left, 46, 47, 63, 65, 76, 80, 84, 106, 108, /Mark Winwood 44, /Jacqui Wornell 18, 31, 83, /Polly Wreford 107, 111.

Photodisc 72, 115.

Executive Editor Jane McIntosh
Editor Rachel Lawrence
Executive Art Editor Peter Burt
Designer Rita Wüthrich
Picture Researcher Zoë Holtermann
Production Controller Jo Sim
Index compiled by Indexing Specialists